HOW NOT TO DIE

IKIGAL: THE JAPANESS SECRET TO A LONG AND HAPPY LIFE

BY

Héctor Greger M.D.

o

Table of Content

INTRODUCTION

IKIGAI: A MYSTERIOUS WORD

IKIGAI

CHAPTER 1

THE ART OF STAYING YOUNG WHILE GROWING OLD

CHAPTER 2

ANTIAGING SECRETS

LITTLE THINGS THAT ADD UP TO A LONG AND HAPPY LIFE

CHAPTER 3

FROM LOGOTHERAPY TO *IKIGAI*

HOW TO LIVE LONGER AND BETTER BY FINDING YOUR PURPOSE

FIGHT FOR YOURSELF

CHAPTER 4

FIND FLOW IN EVERYTHING YOU DO

HOW TO TURN WORK AND FREE TIME INTO SPACES FOR GROWTH

The Seven Conditions for Achieving Flow

CHAPTER 5

MASTERS OF LONGEVITY

Words Of Wisdom From The Longest-Living People In The World

CHAPTER 6

LESSONS FROM JAPAN'S CENTENARIANS

Traditions And Proverbs For Happiness And Longevity

CHAPTER 7

THE *IKIGAI* DIET

What the world's longest-living people eat and drink

CHAPTER 8

GENTLE MOVEMENTS, LONGER LIFE

As Easy as Getting out of Your Chair

Tai chi

CHAPTER 9

RESILIENCE AND *WABI-SABI*

How To Face Life's Challenges Without Letting Stress And Worry Age You

INTRODUCTION

Ikigai: A Mysterious Word

This book was inspired on a rainy night in Tokyo, when its authors met for the first time in one of the city's tiniest bars.

Due to the vast distance separating Barcelona from the capital of Japan, we had only ever read each other's writing; however, we had never actually met. Then, a mutual acquaintance put us in touch, beginning a friendship that eventually led to this project and appears destined to last forever.

The following time we met, a year later, we were strolling through a park in downtown Tokyo when we started talking about Western psychological trends, particularly **logotherapy,** which aids people in discovering their life's purpose.

We noted that despite the fact that people continue to look for meaning in their work and daily lives, Viktor Frankl's logotherapy had fallen out of favor among working therapists who preferred other schools of psychology. We ponder queries like: What is the purpose of my life?

Is it enough just to live longer, or should I strive for something more?

Why do some people know what they want and have a zest for life, while others are befuddled?

Ikigai

The mysterious word **ikigai** came up at some point during our conversation. This Japanese concept, which roughly translates as "the happiness of always being busy," is similar to logotherapy, but it goes a step further. It also appears to be one explanation for the Japanese's extraordinary longevity, particularly on the island of Okinawa, where there are 24.55 people over the age of 100 for every 100,000 inhabitants—far more than the global average.

The ikigai that shapes their lives, according to those who study why the inhabitants of this island in the south of Japan live longer than people anywhere else on the planet, is one of the keys, along with a healthy diet, a simple life in the outdoors, green tea, and the subtropical climate (its average temperature is similar to that of Hawaii).

During our research, we realized that there is not a single book in the fields of psychology or self improvement that aims to bring this philosophy to the West.

Is ikigai the reason Okinawa has the highest number of centenarians? How does it motivate people to keep going until the end? What is the key to living a long, happy life?

Further research revealed that Ogimi, a small rural town on the island's north coast with a population of 3,000, has the highest life expectancy in the world, earning it the nickname the Village of Longevity.

The majority of Japan's shikuwasa—a fruit resembling a lime and packed with extraordinary antioxidant power—comes from Okinawa. Could that be the key to Ogimi's long life? Or is it the quality of the water used to make the tea made from Moringa?

We made the decision to travel to Japan to learn the secrets of the country's centenarians. Our cameras and recording equipment were ready when we arrived in the village, where people still speak an ancient dialect and follow an animist religion that includes long-haired forest spirits known as bunagaya. As soon as we got there, we could feel the incredible friendliness of the locals, who were giggling and making jokes nonstop among the verdant hills fed by crystal clear waters.

As we interviewed the town's senior citizens, we realized that something far more powerful than its natural resources was at work: an uncommon joy flows from its people and guides them through the long and pleasurable journey of their lives.

Again, the mysterious ikigai.

But what precisely is it? How do you obtain it?

It never stopped surprising us that this haven of nearly eternal life was located in Okinawa, where two hundred thousands innocent lives were murdered at the end of WWII. Okinawans, on the other hand, live by the principle of ichariba chode, a local expression that means "treat everyone like a brother, even if you've never met them before."

It turns out that one of the secrets to Ogimi's residents' happiness is a sense of belonging to a community. They practice yuimaaru, or teamwork, from an early age and are thus accustomed to assisting one another.

Nurturing friendships, eating light, getting enough rest, and engaging in regular, moderate exercise are all important components of good health, but it is their ikigai that drives these centenarians to continue celebrating birthdays and cherishing each new day.

The goal of this book is to reveal the secrets of Japan's centenarians while also equipping you with the tools to discover your own ikigai.

Since people who find their ikigai have everything they require for a long and happy life.

Best wishes!

CHAPTER 1

THE ART OF STAYING YOUNG WHILE GROWING OLD

WHAT IS YOUR REASON FOR BEING?

The Japanese believe that everyone has an ikigai, or what a French philosopher might refer to as a raison d'être. Though they carry it within them, some people have already located their ikigai while others are still looking.

Each of us has a hidden ikigai, and it takes perseverance to uncover it. Those who were born on Okinawa, the island that has the most centenarians worldwide, claim that our ikigai is what motivates us to wake up each morning.

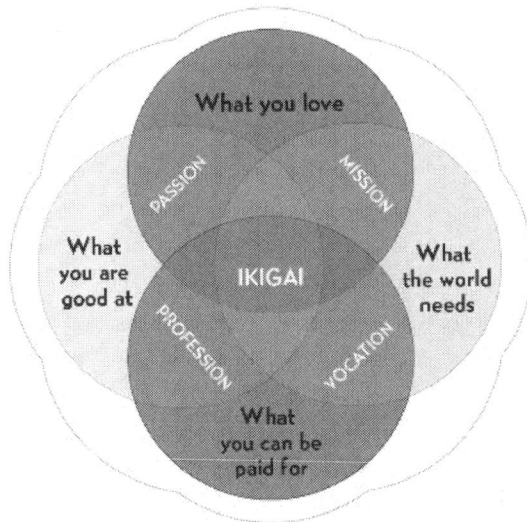

Based on a diagram by Mark Winn

Whatever you do, don't retire!

Our lives are made more fulfilling, joyful, and meaningful when we have a clear understanding of our ikigai. This book's goals are to guide you in discovering yours and to share Japanese philosophical insights on the long-term wellbeing of the body, mind, and spirit.

Living in Japan, one unexpected observation is how active people are even after they retire. Many Japanese individuals actually never truly retire; instead, they continue to pursue their passions for as long as their health permits.

In fact, the Japanese language lacks a word for retirement in the sense of permanently leaving the workforce, as it does in the English language. Dan Buettner, a National Geographic reporter who is well-versed in Japanese culture, claims that retirement simply doesn't exist there because of how important having a purpose in life is in that nation.

The island of (almost) eternal youth

According to some studies on longevity, having a strong sense of community and having a defined ikigai are at least as important as following the famedly better and healthier Japanese diet. Recent medical studies of centenarians from Okinawa and other so-called Blue Zones, the places where people live the longest, reveal a number of fascinating facts about these extraordinary people:

- They not only have significantly longer lifespans than the rest of the world's population, but they also experience fewer chronic diseases like cancer and heart disease, as well as inflammatory disorders.

A large number of these centenarians possess enviable levels of vitality and health that are unheard of for people their age elsewhere.

- Their blood tests show less cellular aging-causing free radicals as a result of drinking tea and eating until they are only 80 percent satisfied.

- Menopause symptoms are more mild for women, and higher levels of sexual hormones are retained in both sexes until much later in life.

- Dementia incidence is significantly lower than the global average.

THE CHARACTERS BEHIND *IKIGAI*

The Japanese word ikigai is written as 生き甲斐, which combines 生き the words "life" and 甲斐"to be worthwhile." 甲斐 can be broken down into 甲 the characters, which means 斐"beautiful" or "elegant," and, which means "armor," "number one," and "to be the first" (to enter battle, taking the initiative as a leader).

Research unmistakably shows that the Okinawans' emphasis on ikigai gives every day a sense of purpose and is crucial to their health and longevity, even though we will discuss each of these findings throughout the course of the book.

The Five Blue Zones

The Blue Zones of the world are led by Okinawa. Women in Okinawa, more than anywhere else in the world, live longer and experience fewer diseases. In his book The Blue Zones, Dan Buettner identifies and examines five geographic areas. They are:

1. **Japan's Okinawa (especially the northern part of the island).**

The locals eat a lot of tofu and vegetables, usually on small plates. The moai, or close-knit group of friends (see page 15), in addition to their ikigai philosophy, is crucial to their longevity.

2. **Italy's Sardinia (specifically the provinces of Nuoro and Ogliastra).**

On this island, residents regularly drink one or two glasses of wine and eat a lot of vegetables. The community's sense of cohesiveness is another element directly related to longevity, just like in Okinawa.

3. Californian city Loma Linda.

One of the oldest populations in the country, Seventh-day Adventists, were the subject of research.

4. Costa Rica's Nicoya Peninsula.

Locals are remarkably active even after turning 90; many of the area's senior citizens have no trouble rising at 5:30 a.m. to work in the fields.

5. Greece's Ikaria.

This island near the Turkish coast is known as the Island of Long Life because one in three of its residents is over 90 years old (as opposed to less than 1% of the population of the United States). A way of life that dates back to 500 BC appears to be the local trade secret.

In the following chapters, we will look at several factors that tend to be the keys to longevity and are found in Blue Zones around the world, with a focus on

Okinawa and its so-called Village of Longevity. But first, it's worth noting that three of these regions are islands, where resources can be hard to obtain and communities must rely on one another.

Helping others may be an ikigai strong enough to keep many people alive.

Diet, exercise, finding a purpose in life (an ikigai), and forming strong social ties—that is, having a large circle of friends and good family relations—are the keys to longevity, according to scientists who have studied the five Blue Zones.

In order to reduce stress, members of these communities have good time management skills, eat little meat or processed food, and consume alcohol in moderation.

They don't engage in vigorous activity, but they do move every day by going on walks and working in their vegetable gardens. The Blue Zones population prefers to walk over driving. The activity that almost all of them engage in daily low-intensity movement is gardening.

The 80 Percent Secret

One of the most widely used phrases in Japan is "Hara hachi bu," which is uttered before or after eating and roughly translates to "Fill your belly to 80%." We should not eat until we are full, according to ancient wisdom. For this reason, Okinawans stop eating when they feel that their stomachs are 80 percent full rather than overeating and taxing their bodies with protracted digestive processes that speed up cellular oxidation.

Of course, there is no accurate way to determine whether your stomach is 80 percent full. This proverb's message is that we should stop eating as soon as we start to feel full. The apple pie after lunch, the extra side dish, and the snack we eat even though we know deep down that we don't really need them will all make us happy in the moment, but they won't make us happy in the long run.

The presentation of the food is also crucial. Japanese people typically eat less because their meals are served on numerous small plates. Four of the five plates in a typical Japanese restaurant meal are quite small, while the main dish is slightly larger. Even though it appears that you will eat a lot when you have five plates in front of you, you typically end up feeling only slightly hungry. This is one of the factors that contribute to Westerners in Japan typically maintaining a trim physique.

Okinawans have a body mass index between 18 and 22, compared to 26 or 27 in the United States, and consume an average of 1,800 to 1,900 calories daily, according to recent nutritionist studies.

The Okinawan diet is high in tofu, sweet potatoes, fish (three times per week), and vegetables (roughly 11 ounces per day). We will learn which nutritious, antioxidant-rich foods make up this 80 percent in the chapter on nutrition.

Moai: Connected For Life

In Okinawa, it is characteristic for neighbors to become close friends. A moai is a loose association of people who share interests and watch out for one another. Serving the community becomes a large part of many people's ikigai.

The moai has its roots in difficult times when farmers would gather to exchange best practices and support one another as they struggled with small harvests.

A moai's members contribute a predetermined amount each month. They are able to partake in gatherings, meals, matches of go and shogi (Japanese chess), as well as any other shared interests, thanks to this payment.

If there is money left over after paying for activities, one member (chosen on a rotating basis) receives a predetermined sum from the surplus. Being a part of a moai aids in preserving both emotional and monetary stability in this way. A moai member who is having financial difficulties may be granted an advance from the group's savings. The specifics of each moai's accounting procedures vary depending on the group and its financial capabilities, but the sense of support and belonging gives the individual a sense of security and lengthens life expectancy.

• • •

Following this brief overview of the subjects covered in this book, we examine a few factors that contribute to early aging in contemporary society before examining various aspects of ikigai.

CHAPTER 2

ANTIAGING SECRETS

Little Things That Add Up To A Long And Happy Life

Aging's Escape Velocity

Our ability to extend life has allowed us to do so for more than a century, adding an average of 0.3 years annually. What would occur though if we had the technology to increase life expectancy by a year a year? Theoretically, after reaching the "escape velocity" of aging, we would become biological immortals.

Aging's Escape Velocity and the Rabbit

Consider a sign in the far future with a number on it representing the age of your death. Every year that you live brings you closer to the sign. You die when you reach the sign.

Consider a rabbit carrying the sign and walking into the future. The rabbit is half a year away for every year you live. You will eventually reach the rabbit and die.

But what if the rabbit could walk one year for each year of your life? You'd never be able to catch the rabbit, and thus you'd never die.

Our technology is the speed with which the rabbit walks to the future. The more we advance technology and our understanding of our bodies, the faster we will be able to make the rabbit walk.

The escape velocity of aging is the point at which the rabbit walks at one year per year or faster and we become immortal.

Future-focused scientists like Ray Kurzweil and Aubrey de Grey assert that we will achieve this escape velocity within a few decades. Some scientists are less upbeat and believe that no matter how much technology we develop, we will eventually reach a maximum age that we will not be able to surpass. For instance, according to some biologists, our cells stop regenerating after 120 years.

Active Mind, Youthful Body

The adage "a sound mind in a sound body" (mens sana in corpore sano) is filled with great wisdom. It serves as a reminder that the health of the body and mind are interrelated and that each is significant. It has been demonstrated that one of the most important aspects of staying young is maintaining an active, adaptable mind.

A young mind encourages you to lead a healthy lifestyle that will delay the effects of aging.

Lack of mental exercise is bad for us because it weakens our neurons and neural connections, which affects our ability to respond to our environment. This is similar to how lack of physical exercise affects our bodies and mood.

This is why it's crucial to exercise your brain.

Shlomo Breznitz, an Israeli neuroscientist, is one of the forerunners in promoting mental exercise. He contends that the brain needs a lot of stimulation to stay in shape. In an interview with Eduard Punset for the Spanish television program Redes, he said the following:

> *What is best for someone and what they want to do are at odds with one another. This is due to the fact that individuals, especially older individuals, prefer to behave in a particular way. The difficulty arises when the brain no longer needs to think because of established habits. Automatically, things get done effectively and quickly, frequently in a very beneficial way. The only way to overcome this tendency to stick to routines is to present the brain with fresh information.*

When the brain is exposed to new information, it renews itself and forms new connections. This is why it is so crucial to expose yourself to change, even if doing so causes you to experience some anxiety.

Scientific evidence supports the benefits of mental training. In their book Maximum Brainpower: Challenging the Brain for Health and Wisdom, Collins Hemingway and Shlomo Breznitz assert that mental training has numerous advantages: "By doing a certain task for the first time, you begin exercising your brain," he writes. "And while it initially seems very challenging, the training is already effective as you learn how to do it. The second time, you realize that because you're getting better at it, it's actually easier to do than the first. This has a wonderful impact on how someone feels. It is a transformation in and of itself that impacts not only the outcomes but also the person's self-image.

It may sound a little formal to describe something as a "mental workout," but simply interacting with others—playing a game, for instance—offers fresh stimuli and mitigates the depression that can result from solitude.

While we are still in our twenties, our neurons begin to deteriorate. However, intellectual activity, curiosity, and a desire to learn slow this process down. Playing games, interacting with others, dealing with novel situations, learning something new every day, and dealing with new situations all appear to be crucial mental antiaging techniques. A more upbeat outlook in this regard will also result in greater mental advantages.

Stress: Accused Of Killing Longevity

Many people appear older than they actually are. Stress has a significant impact on the causes of premature aging, according to research, because it causes the body to deteriorate more quickly in times of stress. After researching this deteriorating process, the American Institute of Stress came to the conclusion that stress is to blame for the majority of health issues.

The issue is that while this reaction neutralizes dangerous substances, it also damages healthy cells, causing them to senescence early.

In a related study, the University of California compared samples from women with healthy children and low levels of stress to samples from 39 women who experienced high levels of stress as a result of the illness of one of their children. They discovered that stress accelerates cellular aging by weakening telomeres, which have an impact on cell regeneration and how our cells age. The study found that stress has a direct correlation with how quickly cells age.In a study, conducted by researchers at the Heidelberg University Hospital, a young physician was put through a stressful job interview while also being required to complete difficult math problems for 30 minutes. They then took a sample of blood. What they found was that his antibodies had responded to stress similarly to how they respond to pathogens, activating the immune response-triggering proteins.

How Does Stress Work?

People live in a frenetic pace and almost constant state of competition today. Stress is a normal reaction to the information the body is receiving at this fever pitch as potentially dangerous or problematic.

Theoretically, this is a good response because it aids in our survival in hostile environments. We have used this reaction throughout the course of our evolution to deal with challenging circumstances and to escape predators.

When we hear an alarm, our brain's neurons trigger the pituitary gland, which releases hormones that cause the release of corticotropin, which is then transported throughout the body by the sympathetic nervous system. Then adrenaline and cortisol are released from the adrenal gland. Cortisol increases the release of dopamine and blood glucose, which is what gets us "charged up" and enables us to face challenges. Adrenaline increases our respiratory rate, pulse, and muscle readiness, preparing the body to react to perceived danger.

Cave Dwellers	Modern Humans
Were relaxed most of the time.	Work most of the time and are alert to any and all threats.
Felt stress only in very specific situations.	Are online or waiting for notifications from their cell phones twenty-four hours a day.
The threats were real: A predator could end their lives at any moment.	The brain associates the ping of a cell phone or an e-mail notification with the threat of a predator.
High doses of cortisol and adrenaline at moments of danger kept the body healthy.	Low doses of cortisol flow constantly through the body, with implications for a range of health problems, including adrenal fatigue and chronic fatigue syndrome.

In moderation, these procedures are advantageous because they aid us in overcoming obstacles in daily life. Nevertheless, it is obvious that the stress that modern humans experience is unhealthy.

Over time, stress has a degenerative effect. The neurons involved in memory are impacted by a protracted state of emergency, which also inhibits the release of some hormones that, when absent, can lead to depression. Irritability, insomnia, anxiety, and high blood pressure are some of its side effects.

In light of this, we should modify our high-stress lifestyles in order to prevent the early aging of our bodies, even though challenges are good for keeping mind and body active.

Be Mindful About Reducing Stress

Stress is a readily recognisable condition that not only causes anxiety but is also highly psychosomatic, affecting everything from our digestive system to our skin, whether or not the threats we perceive are real.

This is why mindfulness practice is highly recommended by many experts in order to avoid the negative effects that stress has on us.

This stress-reduction technique's main tenet is self-awareness: noticing our reactions, even if they are conditioned by habit, in order to be fully aware of them. By doing so, we can focus on the present moment and control thoughts that have a propensity to spiral out of control.

"We must learn to deactivate the autopilot that is guiding us in a circular motion. Everyone has acquaintances who like to munch while on the phone or watching the news. When you ask someone if the omelet they just ate contained onions, they are unable to answer, claims Roberto Alcibar, who gave up his fast-paced lifestyle to pursue his certification as a mindfulness instructor after experiencing a period of extreme stress due to illness.

Through meditation, which helps us sift through the information that comes to us from the outside world, one can achieve a state of mindfulness. Additionally, yoga, body scans, and breathing exercises can help you achieve it.

While developing mindfulness requires a gradual training process, with some practice we can learn to completely focus our minds, which lowers stress and extends our lives.

A little stress is good for you

Low levels of stress have been shown to be advantageous, whereas sustained, intense stress is known to be detrimental to longevity and to both mental and physical health.

Dr. Howard S. Friedman, a psychology professor at the University of California, Riverside, found that people who maintained a low level of stress, who overcame obstacles and gave their all to their work in order to succeed, lived longer than those who chose a more relaxed lifestyle and retired earlier. This was the result of his more than 20 years of observation of a group of test subjects. From this, he deduced that a small amount of stress is beneficial because people who experience little stress tend to form healthier habits, smoke less, and consume less alcohol.

As a result, it is not surprising that many of the supercentenarians—those who live to be 110 or more—that we will meet in this book talk about having led active lives and working into their senior years.

A Lot Of Sitting Will Age You

The increase in sedentary behavior, particularly in the Western world, has contributed to many illnesses like obesity and hypertension, which have an impact on longevity.

Too much time spent sitting down at work or home affects one's ability to breathe and move around, as well as their appetite and desire to engage in physical activity. Sedentary lifestyles can cause hypertension, unbalanced eating, heart disease, osteoporosis, and even some types of cancer. Recent research has linked a lack of exercise to immune system cells' progressive telomere distortion, which in turn ages those cells and the organism as a whole.

This is a problem that affects people of all ages, not just adults. It's crucial to adopt a healthy, active lifestyle early on because inactive children have high rates of obesity and all the related health problems and risks.

Being less sedentary is simple; all it takes is some effort and minor routine adjustments. We only need to incorporate a few components into our regular routines to access a more active lifestyle that improves our overall health:

- Walk at least 20 minutes each day, whether it's to work or just for exercise.
- Instead of using an escalator or elevator, use the stairs. Along with other benefits, this is good for your muscles, respiratory system, and posture.
- Avoid watching television for extended periods of time by engaging in social or recreational activities.
- You'll have more nutrients in your system and less of an urge to snack if you swap out your junk food for fruit.
- Sleep the recommended amount. Anywhere from seven to nine hours is ideal, but any more makes us drowsy.
- Play with children or with animals, join a sports team, or both. This improves self-

esteem and stimulates the mind in addition to strengthening the body.

- Be aware of your daily activities to spot unhealthy routines and swap them out for more constructive ones.

We can start to renew our bodies and minds and lengthen our lives by implementing these small changes.

A Model's Best-Kept Secret

Even though we experience both physical and mental aging, one of the things that tells us the most about a person's age is their skin, which changes in texture and color depending on processes occurring below the surface. Most professional models assert that the night before a fashion show, they get between nine and ten hours of sleep. As a result, their skin appears taut, wrinkle-free, and radiantly healthy.

Because we produce the hormone melatonin while we sleep, which is a hormone that naturally exists in our bodies, science has demonstrated that sleep is a crucial antiaging tool. It plays a part in our sleep and waking cycles and is produced by the pineal gland from the neurotransmitter serotonin in accordance with our diurnal and nocturnal rhythms.

Melatonin, a potent antioxidant, prolongs our lives and provides the following advantages:

- The immune system is strengthened by it.
- It has a component that guards against cancer.
- It encourages the body to produce insulin naturally.
- It delays Alzheimer's disease's onset.
- It protects against heart disease and osteoporosis.

Melatonin is an excellent ally in maintaining youth due to all of these factors. However, it should be noted that after the age of 30, melatonin production declines. This can be made up for by:

- consuming more calcium and maintaining a balanced diet.
- getting some sun each day, but not too much.
- getting sufficient sleep.
- avoiding things like stress, alcohol, tobacco, and caffeine, all of which interfere with getting a good night's sleep and deprive us of melatonin.

Experts are investigating whether melatonin production can be artificially stimulated to slow down the aging process, which would support the idea that we already possess the key to longevity.

Antiaging Attitudes

The body's aging process and how quickly it ages are greatly influenced by the mind. The majority of medical professionals concur that maintaining an active mind, a crucial component of ikigai, and resisting giving in to challenges throughout life are the keys to keeping the body young.

A positive view and intense emotional awareness are two dispositional traits shared by the people who live the longest, according to a study from Yeshiva University. In other words, those who are able to control their emotions and approach problems with a positive attitude are already well on their way to a long life.

A stoic attitude-Being calm in the face of adversity—which reduces anxiety and stress and stabilizes behavior—can also help you stay young. The longer life spans of some cultures with leisurely, deliberate lifestyles are evidence of this.

Many centenarians and supercentenarians share characteristics: they lived full lives that were occasionally challenging, but they learned how to approach these difficulties with a positive attitude and not be overcome by the challenges they faced.

Alexander Imich, who at age 111 became the oldest man alive, was aware that other factors also played a role in his longevity. "The life you live is equally or more important for longevity," he said in an interview with Reuters following his induction into the Guinness Book of Records in 2014.

An Ode To Longevity

A woman who was approaching 100 years old performed the following song for us while we were visiting Ogimi, the village that holds the Guinness record for longevity, in a mix of Japanese and the local dialect:

To live a long and healthy life, savor each bite of everything you eat. early to bed, early to rise, and then go for a walk.We enjoy the journey and live each day in peace.

To live a long and healthy life, All of our friends get along well with us.

Winter, fall, and springWe happily take pleasure in each season.

The trick is to not be preoccupied with the age of the fingers; Your fingers will continue to work if you keep going, and you'll live to be 100.

Now that we have reached the next chapter, we can use our fingers to turn the page and examine the connection between finding our life's purpose and living a long life.

CHAPTER 3

FROM LOGOTHERAPY TO *IKIGAI*

How To Live Longer And Better By Finding Your Purpose

What Is Logotherapy?

When asked to summaries his school of psychology in a single sentence by a colleague, Viktor Frankl responded, "Well, in logotherapy the patient sits up straight and has to listen to things that, on occasion, are hard to hear." He had just heard his colleague describe psychoanalysis in the following way: "In psychoanalysis, the patient lies down on a couch and tells you things that, on occasion, are hard to say."

Why don't you commit suicide? was one of the first questions Frankl would ask his patients, according to him. Usually, the patient came up with valid justifications not to and was able to continue. So what does logotherapy accomplish?

The answer is pretty obvious: It aids in discovering reasons to live.

In order to address their neuroses, logotherapy encourages patients to consciously determine their life's purpose. Then, their desire to fulfill their destiny drives them to move forward, freeing their minds from the past and overcoming any challenges they come across.

Something to Live For

In a study he conducted in his Vienna clinic, Frankl discovered that between patients and staff, about 80% thought that people needed a reason to live, and about 60% thought they had someone or something in their lives that was worth dying for.

The Search For Meaning

The search for purpose became a personal, driving force that allowed Frankl to achieve his goals. The process of logotherapy can be summarized in these five steps:

1. One experiences emptiness, frustration, or anxiety.
2. The therapist helps him understand that his desire for a purposeful life is what is driving those feelings.
3. The patient finds his purpose in life (at that particular point in time).
4. The patient chooses whether to accept or reject that destiny of his own free will.
5. He overcomes challenges and sorrows thanks to his newly discovered passion for life.

Frankl himself was willing to sacrifice everything for his beliefs and ideals. "Everything can be taken from a man except one thing: the last of the human freedoms—to choose one's attitude in any given set of circumstances, to choose one's own way," he wrote after his time as an Auschwitz prisoner. He had to experience it on his own, without assistance, and it served as an inspiration for the rest of his life.

Ten Differences Between Psychoanalysis And Logotherapy

Psychoanalysis	Logotherapy
The patient reclines on a couch, like a patient.	The patient sits facing the therapist, who guides him or her without passing judgment.
Is retrospective: It looks to the past.	Looks toward the future.
Is introspective: It analyzes neuroses.	Does not delve into the patient's neuroses.
The drive is toward pleasure.	The drive is toward purpose and meaning.
Centers on psychology.	Includes a spiritual dimension.
Works on psychogenic neuroses.	Also works on noogenic, or existential, neuroses.
Analyzes the unconscious origin of conflicts (instinctual dimension).	Deals with conflicts when and where they arise (spiritual dimension).
Limits itself to the patient's instincts.	Also deals with spiritual realities.
Is fundamentally incompatible with faith.	Is compatible with faith.

Seeks to reconcile conflicts and satisfy impulses and instincts.	Seeks to help the patient find meaning in his life and satisfy his moral principles.

Fight For Yourself

When our life has no purpose or when our life's purpose is distorted, existential frustration results. But in Frankl's opinion, there is no need to consider this frustration an aberration or a sign of neurosis; rather, it can be a good thing—a driver of change.

In contrast to other forms of therapy, logotherapy points of view this frustration as spiritual anguish—a natural and beneficial phenomenon that drives those who experience it to seek a cure, whether alone or with the assistance of others, and in doing so, to find greater satisfaction in life. It enables them to alter their own fate.

When someone needs assistance with this, with finding their life's purpose and later with resolving conflicts so they can continue moving toward their goal, logotherapy comes into play. Frankl quotes one of Nietzsche's well-known aphorisms from Man's Search for Meaning: "He who has a why to live for can bear with almost any how."

Frankl held the opinion that the tension that results from contrasting our current accomplishments with our long-term goals is necessary for our health, based on his own experiences. The challenge we need is something we can strive to overcome by using all the tools at our disposal, not a peaceful existence.

Contrarily, existential crisis is typical of contemporary societies where people follow orders or the behavior of others rather than their own desires. They frequently try to bridge the gap between what is expected of them and what they want for themselves by numbing their senses, gaining economic power, or engaging in physical pleasure. It might even result in suicide.

For instance, Sunday neurosis is when someone becomes aware of how empty they are on the inside because they are not subject to the responsibilities and commitments of the workweek. He must come up with a solution. He needs to identify his ikigai—his reason for getting out of bed—above all else.

"I Feel Empty Inside"

Frankl's team discovered that 55% of the patients they spoke with at the Vienna Polyclinic Hospital were going through some sort of existential crisis.

Better Living Through Logotherapy: A Few Key Ideas

- In contrast to what Sartre asserted, we discover the meaning of our lives.
- Every one of us has a special purpose for existing, which can change over time.

- In the same way that worrying frequently results in exactly what was feared, giving a desire too much thought (also known as "hyper-intention") can prevent it from materializing.
- Positive cycles can be broken and anxiety can be decreased with humor.
- Every one of us is capable of both good and bad deeds. Our decisions, not our circumstances, determine which side of the equation we fall on.

We will examine four cases from Frankl's own practice in the pages that follow in order to better understand the pursuit of meaning and purpose.

Case Study: Viktor Frankl

Psychiatrists confirmed that the prisoners with the best chances of surviving in German concentration camps, as well as in those that would later be built in Japan and Korea, were those who had goals outside the camp and who felt a strong need to escape from there alive. In Frankl's case, he realized he had been the first client of his own practice after being freed and successfully founding the logotherapy school.

Frankl persisted because he had a target to reach. His manuscript, ready for publication, contained all the theories and research he had gathered over the course of his career when he arrived at Auschwitz. To the extent that over the years, and particularly when he contracted typhus, he would jot down passages and key words from the lost work on any scrap of paper he found, this need drove him and gave his life meaning amid the constant horror and uncertainty of the concentration camp

Case Study: The American Diplomat

An important North American diplomat visited Frankl to continue a course of treatment he had begun in the United States five years earlier. The diplomat responded that he hated his job and the international policies of his country, which he had to uphold, when Frankl asked him why he had initially begun therapy. In order for his government and his job, both of which served as representations of the paternal figure, to appear less unfavorable, his American psychoanalyst, with whom he had been consulting for years, insisted that he make peace with his father. Frankl, however, convinced the diplomat in a relatively short number of sessions that his dissatisfaction stemmed from his desire to pursue a different line of work, and the diplomat ended his treatment with that in mind.

The former diplomat revealed to Frankl five years later that he had been working in a different field during that time and was content.

The man, in Frankl's opinion, not only didn't require all those years of psychoanalysis, but he couldn't even be regarded as a "patient" in need of therapy. He was simply looking for a new reason for living, and as soon as he did, his life began to mean more.

Case Study: The Suicidal Mother

The mother of a boy who had passed away at age eleven was brought into Frankl's clinic after she and her other son attempted suicide. He did believe his life had a purpose, and if their mother killed them both, it would prevent him from achieving his goals. It was this other son, who had been paralyzed since birth, who prevented her from carrying out her plan.

In a group discussion, the woman told her tale. To assist her, Frankl asked another woman to picture herself as an elderly, affluent, but childless woman lying on her deathbed. The woman insisted that she would have felt her life had been a failure in that situation.

The suicidal mother was instructed to complete the same exercise while visualizing herself on her deathbed; as she did so, she looked back and realized that she had done everything she could for her children—for both of them. She had provided a good life for her paralyzed son, and he had grown into a decent and contented adult. She continued, sobbing, "As for myself, I can look back on my life with peace because I can say that my life was full of meaning and I have tried hard to live it fully; I have done my best—I have done my best for my son. I can say that my life was full of meaning. My life has been successful!

The suicidal mother discovered the meaning that her life already had even though she was not aware of it by visualizing herself on her deathbed and looking back.

Case Study: The Grief-Stricken Doctor

An elderly doctor sought Frankl's assistance because he was struggling to recover from the severe depression he had experienced following the death of his wife two years earlier.

Frankl questioned him about what would have happened if he had passed away first, rather than offering advice or discussing his health. The horrified doctor responded that his poor wife would have suffered greatly and that it would have been terrible for her. Frankl then retorted, "You see, doctor? You have spared her from all that suffering, but you must live and mourn her as a result.

The physician stopped speaking after that. He took the therapist's hand and walked out of Frankl's office in peace. In the place of his cherished wife, he was able to endure the suffering. His existence now had meaning.

Morita Therapy

Shoma Morita developed his own purpose-centered therapy in Japan during the same decade as logotherapy—a few years earlier, in fact. Posttraumatic stress disorder, obsessive-compulsive disorder, and neurosis were all successfully treated with it

Shoma Morita was not only a psychotherapist but also a Zen Buddhist, and his therapy had a profound spiritual impact on Japan.

The goal of many Western therapeutic approaches is to manage or alter the patient's emotions. In the West, we have a propensity to think that our thoughts affect our feelings, which in turn affect our actions. Contrarily, since patients' actions will alter their feelings, Morita therapy focuses on teaching patients to accept their emotions without attempting to control them.

Morita therapy aims to "create" new emotions based on actions in addition to accepting the patient's current emotions. These emotions, in Morita's opinion, are learned through practice and experience.

Morita therapy teaches us to accept our desires, anxieties, fears, and worries and let them go rather than trying to get rid of the symptoms. It is best to be rich and kind when it comes to feelings, according to Morita, who writes about this in his book Morita Therapy and the True Nature of Anxiety-Based Disorders.

The following parable was used by Morita to illustrate the concept of letting go of unfavorable emotions: If a donkey is tied to a post with a rope, it will keep walking around the post in an effort to break free, only to become more immobilized and attached to the post. The same holds true for those who struggle with obsessive thinking, who find themselves further enmeshed in their own misery when they make an effort to flee their anxieties and discomfort.

The Basic Principles Of Morita Therapy

Embrace your feelings and thoughts: If we experience obsessive thoughts, we shouldn't attempt to suppress or control them. They get more intense if we do. The Zen master used to say, "If we try to get rid of one wave with another, we end up with an infinite sea," in reference to human emotions. Our feelings don't originate from us; we simply have to accept them when they do. Greeting them is the key. Morita compared emotions to the weather, saying that we can only observe them and not predict or control them. He frequently used the words of the Vietnamese monk Thich Nhat Hanh, who would greet solitude by saying, "Hello. How are you doing today? I will look after you if you will sit with me.

Follow the right course of action: Instead of concentrating on treating the symptoms, we should wait for recovery to occur naturally. Instead, we ought to concentrate on the here and now, and, if we are in pain, on accepting that pain. Above all, we must refrain from overthinking the situation. Character is rooted in the things we do, and the therapist's goal is to help the patient develop it so they can handle any situation. Patients receiving Morita therapy are not given explanations; instead, they are given the opportunity to learn from their own actions and activities. In contrast to Western therapies, it doesn't instruct you on how to practice meditation or keep a journal. The patient must learn new things through experience.

Discover what your life's purpose is: While we cannot control our emotions, we can always choose how we will behave. Because of this, we should be clear about our goals and constantly remember Morita's maxim: "What do we need to be doing right now? What steps ought we to take? The secret to doing this is having the courage to look within to discover your ikigai.

The Four Phases Of Morita Therapy

Morita's original treatment, which lasts between fifteen and twenty-one days, is divided into the following stages:

Isolation and rest (five to seven days): The patient rests in a room with no outside stimulation during the first week of treatment. No speaking, reading, television, family, or friends. The patient is left with nothing but his thoughts. He receives frequent visits from the therapist, who makes an effort to avoid interacting with him as much as possible, and spends the majority of the day lying down. The therapist simply suggests to the patient to keep observing the ups and downs of his emotions as he lies there. The patient is prepared to advance to the next phase of therapy when he becomes bored and wants to resume doing things.

Light occupational therapy (five to seven days) : At this point, the patient works silently through monotonous tasks. One of them is writing down his thoughts and emotions in a journal. After a week of isolation, the patient ventures outside for nature walks and breathing exercises. He also starts engaging in basic activities like gardening, painting, and drawing. The only person the patient is permitted to speak to at this point is the therapist.

Occupational therapies (five to seven days): At this point, the patient engages in activities that call for movement. Dr. Morita loved to go woodcutting with his patients in the mountains. The patient is also engaged in non-physical tasks, such as writing, painting, or creating ceramics, in addition to physical ones. At this point, the patient can converse with others, but only regarding the tasks at hand.

Returning to social interactions and the "real" world: After leaving the hospital, the patient is reintroduced to society while continuing the meditation and occupational therapy routines they developed while receiving treatment.

Reentering society as a fresh individual, motivated by a purpose, and free from emotional or social constraints is the goal.

Naikan meditation

Morita was a renowned expert in Naikan introspective meditation and a Zen master. He frequently refers to this school in his therapy, which is based on three questions the patient must ask themselves:

What have I received from person X

What have I given to person X?

What problems have I caused person X?

By doing these philosophical ramblings, we stop blaming others for our problems and develop a stronger sense of personal accountability. If you're angry and want to fight, consider it for three days before you do, as Morita advised. The intense desire to fight will naturally subside after three days.

And Now Ikigai

Finding your ikigai, or existential fuel, is the quest that underpins both logotherapy and Morita therapy. You can access this experience without the aid of therapists or spiritual retreats. Once you've located it, all that's left to do is muster the courage and exert the necessary effort to continue down the correct path.

The basic tools you'll need to start down that path will be discussed in the chapters that follow. These include learning to find flow in the activities you've chosen, eating a balanced, mindful diet, engaging in low-intensity exercise, and developing the ability to persevere in the face of challenges. To achieve this, you must acknowledge that although the world is flawed, just like the people who inhabit it, there are still plenty of chances for personal development and success. Are you prepared to give everything you have to your passion and act as if it were the most important thing in the world?

CHAPTER 4

FIND FLOW IN EVERYTHING YOU DO

How To Turn Work And Free Time Into Spaces For Growth

Going With The Flow

Consider skiing down a slope that you enjoy. White sand-like snowpowder rises up on either side of you. The environment is ideal.

You give your complete attention to skiing as well as you can. You are always aware of your best course of action. No past or future exist. There is nothing but now. Your body, your skis, the snow, and your consciousness are all felt as one cohesive entity. There is nothing else on your mind or keeping you from being fully present in the experience. Your ego vanishes, and you merge with your activity.

In his well-known speech "Be water, my friend," Bruce Lee spoke of exactly this sort of experience.

Everybody has experienced how time seems to fly by when they are engaged in an enjoyable activity. As soon as we get started cooking, several hours have already passed. Before we notice the sunset and remember we haven't had dinner, we spend an afternoon reading and losing track of time. When we go surfing, we don't count the number of hours we spend in the water until our muscles hurt the next day.

The complete opposite is also possible. Every minute feels like a lifetime when we have to finish a task we don't want to do, and we are unable to stop checking the time. Put your hand on a hot stove for a minute and it will feel like an hour, according to an adage attributed to Einstein. A beautiful girl makes an hour seem like a minute when you're sitting next to her. Relativity is what that is.

The irony is that we want to finish the task as soon as we can, even though someone else may really enjoy it.

What makes something so enjoyable to us that it causes us to put our worries aside in the process? We are happiest when. We can learn about our ikigai by using these questions.

The Power Of Flow

These issues are also at the center of psychologist Mihaly Csikszentmihalyi's investigation into the sensation of total immersion in our activities. This state, which Csikszentmihalyi termed "flow," was defined as the pleasure, delight, creativity, and process that occur when we are totally immersed in life.

There is no secret to happiness or living your ikigai, but being able to enter this state of flow and experience a "optimal experience" through it is a necessary ingredient.

Instead of allowing ourselves to become engrossed in activities that provide immediate pleasure—like overeating, abusing drugs or alcohol, or stuffing ourselves with chocolate in front of the TV—we must concentrate on increasing the time we spend on activities that transport us into this state of flow.

Flow is "the state in which people are so involved in an activity that nothing else seems to matter; the experience itself is so enjoyable that people will do it even at great cost, for the sheer sake of doing it," according to Csikszentmihalyi in his book Flow: The Psychology of Optimal Experience.

High concentration doses that encourage flow are necessary for everyone, not just creative professionals. A large portion of the time that engineers, chess players, and athletes spend is in pursuits that induce this state.

According to Csikszentmihalyi's research, when in a state of flow, a chess player experiences the same emotions as a mathematician working on a formula or a surgeon carrying out an operation. Csikszentmihalyi, a psychology professor, studied data collected from people all over the world and found that people of all ages and cultures experience flow in the same way. We all enter a state of flow in the same way, whether in Okinawa or New York.

But what transpires in our minds in that circumstance?

When we are in the flow, we are undistractedly focused on a specific task. Our minds are "organized." When we try to do something while thinking about something else, the opposite happens.

There are a number of strategies you can use to increase your chances of achieving flow if you frequently lose focus while working on something you value.

The Seven Conditions for Achieving Flow

The conditions for achieving flow, according to DePaul University researcher Owen Schaffer, are:

1. *Knowing what to do*
2. *Knowing how to do it*
3. *Knowing how well you are doing*
4. *Knowing where to go (where navigation is involved)*
5. *Perceiving significant challenges*
6. *Perceiving significant skills*
7. *Being free from distractions*

Strategy 1: Choose A Difficult Task (But Not Too Difficult!)

The Schaffer model encourages us to take on tasks that are just outside of our comfort zone but that we have a chance of finishing.

There are rules for every activity, including sports and jobs, and adhering to them requires a certain set of abilities. We are likely to become bored if the guidelines for completing a task or achieving a goal are too simple in comparison to our skill level. Too simple a task encourages apathy.

On the other hand, if we set a task that is too challenging for us, we won't be able to finish it, and we'll almost certainly give up along with feeling frustrated.

In order for something to feel challenging to us, it should be in the middle—aligned with our capabilities but just a little bit beyond them. When

Ernest Hemingway said, "Sometimes I write better than I can," he meant this.

We enjoy the feeling of pushing ourselves, so we want to see challenges through to the end. When he said, "To be able to concentrate for a considerable amount of time is essential to difficult achievement," Bertrand Russell echoed this sentiment.

For your upcoming project, graphic designers should learn a new piece of software. Use a new programming language if you're a programmer. Try to include a movement in your next routine if you're a dancer that has long seemed impossible.

Include a little extra, something that forces you to step outside of your comfort zone.

Even something as basic as reading requires following rules and requiring a certain set of skills and knowledge. If we attempt to read a book on quantum mechanics written for physicists who are not ourselves physicists, we will probably give up after a short while. On the other hand, if we already know everything a book has to say, we'll quickly grow bored.

However, if the book is in line with our skills and knowledge and expands on what we already know, we'll become engrossed in it and the time will fly. We are in tune with our ikigai if we are experiencing this pleasure and satisfaction.

Easy	Challenging	Beyond Our Abilities
Boredom	Flow	Anxiety

Strategy 2: Have A Clear, Concrete Objective

Sports, board games, and video games—when played in moderation—are all excellent ways to achieve flow because the goal is usually very clear: While adhering to a clear set of instructions, beat your opponent or your own record.

Unfortunately, the goal isn't always as obvious in these circumstances.

According to a Boston Consulting Group study, employees at multinational corporations' top complaint about their managers is that they fail to "communicate the team's mission clearly," which leaves the staff members in the dark about their goals.

What frequently occurs, especially in large corporations, is that the executives become mired in the minutiae of obsessive planning and develop plans to cover up the fact that they lack a clear goal. It's like sailing out to sea without a destination on your map.

Having a compass that points to a specific goal is far more significant than having a map. In order to navigate our uncertain world, Joi Ito, director of the MIT Media Lab, advises us to use the compass over maps principle. In their book Whiplash: How to Survive Our Faster Future, he and Jeff Howe state, "In an increasingly unpredictable world moving ever more quickly, a detailed map may lead you deep into the woods at an unnecessary high cost. But if you have a good compass, you can always find your way. However, this does not imply that you should set out on your journey with no plan in place. It does, however, imply realizing that even though the road to your destination may not be smooth, you'll arrive there more quickly and effectively than you would have if you had plodded along a predetermined path.

It's crucial to consider our goals before beginning any work, study, or production in business, the creative industries, or education. We should probe ourselves with inquiries like these:

- What is my objective for today's session in the studio?
- How many words am I going to write today for the article coming out next month?
- What is my team's mission?

- How fast will I set the metronome tomorrow in order to play that sonata at an allegro tempo by the end of the week?

In order to achieve flow, having a clear goal is crucial, but once work begins, we must also know how to put the goal aside. We should keep this goal in mind as we travel, but not become fixated on it.

Athletes competing for gold medals at the Olympics are unable to pause to admire the medal. They must flow and be present in the present. They will almost certainly make a mistake at a crucial time and lose the competition if they let themselves get distracted for a moment by thoughts of how happy they'll make their parents when they show them the medal.

This frequently manifests as writer's block. Consider a writer who has three months to complete a novel. The issue is that the writer can't help but become fixated on the goal, even though it is obvious. She gets out of bed each morning with the thought, "I have to write that novel," and immediately gets to work reading the paper and doing the dishes. She expresses frustration every evening and vows to report to work the following day.

When it would have only taken a few minutes to sit down, write the first word, followed by the second to flow with the project and express her ikigai, days, weeks, and even months would have passed with nothing on the page.

Your anxiety will vanish as soon as you take these first, small steps, and you'll experience a pleasant flow in your current activity. A happy man is too content with the present to think about the future, to paraphrase Albert Einstein once more.

Uncertain Objective	Clearly Defined Objective and a Focus on Process	**Obsessive Desire to Achieve a Goal While Ignoring Process**
Confusion; time	**Flow**	Fixation on the

and energy wasted on meaningless tasks		objective rather than getting down to business
Mental block	**Flow**	Mental block

Strategy 3: Concentrate On A Single Task

With so much technology and so many distractions, this is possibly one of the biggest challenges we currently face. While writing an email and watching a YouTube video at the same time, a chat prompt appears and we respond. After our smartphone vibrates in our pocket, we respond to the message and immediately return to our computer to log into Facebook.

Within a matter of minutes, thirty minutes have gone by, and we have forgotten the subject of the email we were writing.

Sometimes we watch a movie while eating dinner and don't appreciate how good the salmon was until we're down to our last bite.

We frequently believe that combining tasks will save us time, but research shows that doing so actually wastes time. Even multitaskers who claim to be efficient are not very effective. They are among the least productive people, in fact.

Even though our brains are capable of processing millions of bits of information per second, they can only do so at any given time. When we say we are multitasking, what we are actually doing is quickly switching between tasks. Unfortunately, we lack the parallel processing capabilities of computers. Instead of concentrating on one task and doing it well, we wind up expending all of our energy switching between them.

The most crucial element in achieving flow may be focusing on one thing at a time.

Csikszentmihalyi affirms that in order to concentrate on a task, we require:

1. To be in a distraction-free environment

2. To have control over what we are doing at every moment

Technology is fantastic as long as we can control it. If it starts to rule us, it's not so good. When writing a research paper, for instance, you might sit down at your computer and use Google to find the data you require. But if you lack discipline, you might find yourself surfing the Internet rather than finishing that paper. Google and the Internet would then have taken control, jerking you out of your zone.

Science has proven that if we ask our brains to switch between tasks frequently, we waste time, commit more errors, and remember less of what we've done.

Our generation is characterized as experiencing an epidemic of multitasking, according to several studies conducted at Stanford University by Clifford Ivar Nass. In one such study, hundreds of students' behavior was examined, and they were divided into groups according to how many activities they tended to engage in simultaneously. The most multitasking-dependent students typically alternated between more than four tasks, such as taking notes while reading a textbook, listening to a podcast, using their smartphone to respond to messages, and occasionally checking their Twitter timeline.

Each class was shown a screen with a number of red and blue arrows. The exercise's goal was to count the red arrows.

At first, all of the students responded correctly right away and with little difficulty. However, as the number of blue arrows increased (while the number of red arrows remained constant; only their position changed), the multitasking students had significant difficulty counting the red arrows in the allotted time or as quickly as the students who did not frequently multitask for one very obvious reason: they became distracted by the blue arrows! The other students' brains were trained to concentrate on a single task—in this case, counting the red arrows and ignoring the blue ones—while the other students' brains were trained to attend to every stimulus, regardless of its significance.

According to other studies, multitasking reduces our productivity by at least 60% and our IQ by more than ten points.

A sample group of more than 4,000 young adults between the ages of twenty and twenty-four who were addicted to their smartphones reported getting less sleep, feeling less part of their school community, and being more likely to exhibit signs of depression, according to a study supported by the Swedish Council for Working Life and Social Research.

Concentrating on a Single Task	Multitasking
Makes achieving flow more	Makes achieving flow

likely	impossible
Increases productivity	Decreases productivity by 60 percent (though it doesn't seem to)
Increases our power of retention	Makes it harder to remember things
Makes us less likely to make mistakes	Makes us more likely to make mistakes
Helps us feel calm and in control of the task at hand	Makes us feel stressed by the sensation that we're losing control, that our tasks are controlling *us*
Causes us to become more considerate as we pay full attention to those around us	Causes us to hurt those around us through our "addiction" to stimuli: always checking our phones, always on social media . . .
Increases creativity	Reduces creativity

What can we do to stop this flow-impeding epidemic from expanding? How can we teach our brains to concentrate on one thing at a time? Here are some suggestions for establishing a distraction-free environment to improve our chances of entering a state of flow and connecting with our ikigai:

- During your first hour of being awake and the hour before you go to sleep, avoid looking at any kind of screen

- Before you reach flow, put your phone away. Nothing is more crucial than the task you have selected to complete at this time. If this seems excessive, turn on the "do not disturb" feature so that only those who are closest to you can get in touch with you in an emergency.

- Establish a day of technological "fasting" every week, perhaps on a Saturday or Sunday, with the exception of e-readers (without Wi-Fi) and MP3 players.

- Consider visiting a cafe without Wi-Fi.

- Only once or twice a day should you read and reply to email. Establish those hours clearly and adhere to them.

- Try the Pomodoro Technique: Get a kitchen timer (some are designed to resemble a pomodoro, or tomato), and resolve to work on one project for the duration of the timer's operation. For each cycle, the Pomodoro Technique suggests 25 minutes of work and 5 minutes of rest, but you can also work for 50 minutes and take 10 minutes off. Choose a pace that works for you; the most crucial thing is to be persistent in finishing each cycle.

- A ritual you enjoy at the start and a reward at the conclusion of your work session

- When you notice that your attention is wandering, practice bringing it back to the present. Whatever will help you regain your focus, such as mindfulness or another type of meditation, a swim or a walk, should be done.

- Work in a place where you won't be interrupted. If you are unable to complete this task at home, visit a library, a coffee shop, or a music studio if it involves playing the saxophone. If your surroundings keep getting in the way, keep looking until you find the proper location.

- Affix a specific location and time to each group of related tasks in each activity. Divide each activity into groups. If you're writing a magazine article, for instance, you might do your research and make notes at home in the morning, write in the library in the afternoon, and edit on the couch in the evening.

- Consider grouping similar tasks together and completing them all at once, such as sending invoices or making calls.

Advantages of Flow	Disadvantages of Distraction
A focused mind	A wandering mind
Living in the present	Thinking about the past and the future
We are free from worry	Concerns about our daily life and the people around us invade our thoughts
The hours fly by	Every minute seems endless

We feel in control	We lose control and fail to complete the task at hand, or other tasks or people keep us from our work
We prepare thoroughly	We act without being prepared
We know what we should be doing at any given moment	We frequently get stuck and don't know how to proceed
Our mind is clear and overcomes all obstacles to the flow of thought	We are plagued by doubts, concerns, and low self-esteem
It's pleasant	It's boring and exhausting
Our ego fades: We are not the ones controlling the activity or task we're doing—the task is leading us	Constant self-criticism: Our ego is present and we feel frustrated

Flow In Japan: Takumis Engineers, Geniuses, And Otakus

What do engineers, inventors, otakus (anime and manga fans), and takumis (craftspeople) have in common? They are all aware of how crucial it is to always follow their ikigai.

Even though some Japanese claim that people in Japan appear to be working harder than they actually are, this is a common stereotype of the country's population. But there is no denying their capacity for total concentration or their persistence when a challenge needs to be overcome. When learning Japanese, one of the first words they encounter is ganbaru, which means "to persevere" or "to stay firm by doing one's best."

Japanese people frequently apply themselves with an intensity that verges on obsession to even the most simple tasks. This can be observed in a variety of settings, such as the "retirees" who meticulously tend to their rice fields in the Nagano mountains or the college students who work the weekend shift at konbini convenience stores. You can see this attention to detail in action in almost every transaction in Japan.

You'll also find that Japan is a treasure trove of traditional craftwork if you enter one of the shops selling handcrafted items in Naha, Kanazawa, or Kyoto. The Japanese people have a special talent for developing   cutting-edge   technology   while preserving handicrafts and traditional methods.

The Art Of The Takumi

Toyota works with "artisans" who can manually create a specific kind of screw. These takumi, or specialists in a specific manual skill, are crucial to Toyota and difficult to replace. Some of them are the sole practitioners of their particular skill, and it doesn't appear that a new generation will take up the mantle.

Another example is turntable needles, which are made almost exclusively in Japan by the last people who still know how to operate the machinery needed to create these precise needles and who are working to pass that knowledge on to their offspring.

On a trip to Kumano, a small town close to Hiroshima, we met a takumi. Working on a photo essay for one of the most well-known makeup brush brands in the West, we were there for the day. The Kumano welcome sign features a mascot holding a sizable brush. The town is filled with small homes and vegetable gardens in addition to the brush factories; as you travel further in, you can see a number of Shinto shrines at the foot of the mountains that surround the town.

Before we realized we still hadn't seen anyone actually putting bristles into the brush heads, we spent hours taking photos in factories full of people in neat rows, each doing a single task, like painting the handles of the brushes or loading boxes of them onto trucks.

The president of one company finally agreed to demonstrate how it was done after we repeatedly asked about this and received the runaround. He asked us to board his car as he led the group of us out of the structure. We parked next to a smaller building after a five-minute drive and went up the stairs. We entered a small room through a door that he had just opened, which was filled with windows that let in lovely natural light.

The room's center was occupied by a woman in a mask. Her eyes were all you could see. She gracefully moved her hands and fingers, sorting the bristles with combs and scissors as she was so intent on picking out individual bristles for the brushes that she was completely unaware of our presence. It was challenging to understand what she was doing because of her swift movements.

She was interrupted by the company president, who informed her that we would be taking pictures while she worked. Although we couldn't see her mouth, the glint in her eye and the upbeat tone in her voice made it clear that she was grinning. As she spoke about her job and responsibilities, she appeared content and proud.

To record her movements, we had to use shutter speeds that were incredibly fast. Together with her tools and the bristles she was sorting, her hands flowed and danced.

Even though she was tucked away in a different building, the company's president claimed that this takumi was one of its most crucial employees. She handled each brush bristle that the company produced.

Steve Jobs In Japan

Steve Jobs, a co-founder of Apple, loved Japan. When he founded Apple, he not only visited the Sony factories in the 1980s and used many of their practices, but he was also mesmerized by Kyoto's simplicity and the high caliber of Japanese porcelain.

But it was a takumi from Toyama named Yukio Shakunaga who used a rare technique called Etchu Seto-yaki who won Steve Jobs's love, not a craftsman from Kyoto.

Jobs learned about a Shakunaga exhibition while in Kyoto. He realized right away that Shakunaga's porcelain was unique in some way. In fact, he returned to the show three times that week and purchased a number of cups, vases, and plates.

Jobs visited Kyoto on numerous occasions throughout his life in search of inspiration and eventually met Shakunaga in person. Jobs reportedly asked him a lot of questions, almost all of which centered on the manufacturing process and the kind of porcelain he employed.

The only artist of his ilk who is familiar with the creation process of porcelain objects from their origins in the mountains to their final form—an authentic takumi—is Shakunaga, who used white porcelain that he extracted himself from mountains in the Toyama prefecture.

Jobs was so moved by this that he thought about traveling to Toyama to see the mountain from which Shakunaga sourced his porcelain, but he changed his mind after learning that it would take him more than four hours to get there by train from Kyoto.

Shakunaga expressed his pride at the iPhone inventor, Steve Jobs, having appreciated his work in a post-mortem interview. He added that Jobs had recently bought a dozen teacups from him. Jobs had requested "a new style," something special. Shakunaga made 150 teacups to fulfill this request while experimenting with new concepts. He sent the twelve best to the Jobs family out of these.

Jobs was fascinated and inspired by Japanese craftspeople, engineers (especially at Sony), philosophy (especially Zen), and cuisine ever since his first visit (especially sushi).

Sophisticated Simplicity

What do Japanese chefs, craftsmen, and engineers have in common with Zen doctrine? attention to detail and simplicity. According to one's ikigai, it is not a simpleton who is lazy but one who is sophisticated and constantly pushing the boundaries of the object, the body and mind, or the cuisine.

The secret to sustaining flow, according to Csikszentmihalyi, is to constantly present a worthwhile challenge to overcome.

We can see another instance of a takumi, this time in the kitchen, in the film Jiro Dreams of Sushi. The book's protagonist, who runs a small sushi restaurant in Tokyo close to the Ginza subway station, has been making sushi every day for more than eighty years. He visits the renowned Tsukiji fish market every day with his son, picking out the best fish to bring back to the restaurant.

One of Jiro's apprentices learning to make tamago is depicted in the documentary (a thin, slightly sweet omelet). He tries desperately to win Jiro's support, but he is unsuccessful. Until he succeeds, he continues to practice for years.

Why won't the apprentice give up? Doesn't he get tired of making eggs every day? No, because he also enjoys making sushi as his ikigai.

Jiro and his son are both talented cooks. When they cook, they enter a state of flow rather than getting bored. When they are in the kitchen, they are completely happy and experiencing ikigai. They've mastered the art of enjoying their work and losing track of time.

They work in a quiet, peaceful environment that enables them to concentrate, in addition to their close relationship, which keeps them motivated each day. They never gave the idea of expanding the business or opening additional locations, even after receiving a three-star rating from Michelin. They only have ten customers at the bar of their little restaurant at any given time. Jiro's family doesn't seek financial gain; instead, they value fair working conditions and fostering an atmosphere where they can freely produce the best sushi in the world.

Jiro starts at "the source" of his work, just like Yukio Shakunaga. Shakunaga searches the mountains for the best porcelain, while he visits the fish market for the best tuna. They become one with the object they are making as soon as they get to work. In Japan, where Shintoism holds that all things, including trees, forests, and objects, contain a kami (spirit or god), this unity with the object that they achieve in a state of flow has a special significance.

It is everyone's responsibility to use nature to give their creations "life" while respecting nature at all times, whether they are chefs, engineers, or artists. The artist flows with the object throughout this process and merges with it. Similar to how someone making ceramics would say the clay has its own life, an ironworker would assert that metal has its own life. The Japanese are skilled at fusing technology and nature together—not as man versus nature, but rather as a fusion of the two.

The Purity Of Ghibli

Some claim that the Shinto value of having a connection to nature is fading away. Hayao Miyazaki, the director of the animated films created by Studio Ghibli, is one of the harshest critics of this loss and is another artist with a clearly defined ikigai.

In almost all of his movies, we see a struggle between fantasy, technology, and nature, which ultimately unites. In his movie Spirited Away, an obese spirit covered in trash who symbolizes river pollution is one of the most moving metaphors.

In Miyazaki's movies, trees and forests have personalities and robots make friends with birds. Miyazaki, who is revered as a national treasure by the government of Japan, is a talented artist who can lose himself entirely in his work. He makes his entire team draw by hand and uses a cell phone from the late 1990s. Even the smallest detail is rendered on paper as he "directs" his movies, achieving flow through drawing rather than a computer. Due to the director's obsession with using traditional methods for almost the entire production process, Studio Ghibli is one of the few places in the world where this is the case.

Those who have been to Studio Ghibli know that it is fairly common to see a lone person working alone in a corner on a given Sunday. The person will be dressed simply and will greet them with an ohayo (hello) without looking up.

Miyazaki is so dedicated to his craft that he frequently spends Sundays in the studio, indulging in the state of flow and prioritizing his ikigai. Visitors are aware that Miyazaki has a short fuse and should never be bothered, especially if he is working on a drawing.

Miyazaki announced his retirement in 2013. The television network NHK produced a documentary depicting him in his final days of employment to honor his retirement. In nearly every scene of the movie, he is drawing. In one scene, several of his coworkers are seen leaving a meeting, and he is sitting in a corner, drawing, completely unconcerned. In another scene, he is seen arriving at work on December 30—a national holiday in Japan—and unlocking Studio Ghibli's doors so he can stay there and draw all day.

Miyazaki is an insatiable artist. Instead of taking a vacation or staying in, he went to Studio Ghibli the day after his "retirement" and sat down to draw. Indecisive about what to say, his coworkers put on their best poker faces. A year later, he declared that he would stop making feature films but would continue to draw up until his passing.

If someone is passionate about their work, can they really retire?

The Recluses

There are scientists and artists all over the world with powerful, distinct ikigais, so this ability is not just possessed by the Japanese. Until they pass away, they continue to do what they love.

Einstein attempted to combine all the forces of the universe in a single theory in his final writing before he closed his eyes forever. He was still working on his passion when he passed away. He claimed that if he hadn't been a physicist, he would have been content as a musician. He enjoyed playing the violin when he wasn't concentrating on physics or math. It gave him endless pleasure to enter a state of flow while working on his formulas or playing music, his two ikigais.

Many of these artists may come across as misanthropic or reclusive, but in reality, they are just trying to protect the moments that make them happy, even if it means sacrificing other aspects of their lives. They are outliers who take the idea of flow and apply it to every aspect of their lives.

The author of the novels Haruki Murakami is another illustration of this type of artist. He only interacts with a small group of friends and only occasionally makes an appearance in Japan's public life.

Artists are aware of how crucial it is to safeguard their territory, maintain control over their surroundings, and be free from outside distractions in order to flow with their ikigai.

Microflow: Enjoying Mundane Tasks

But what happens when we have to, say, clean up after ourselves, mow the lawn, or take care of some paperwork? Is there a way to make these boring tasks enjoyable?

There is a supermarket that still employs elevator operators close to the Shinjuku subway stop, in one of the brain centers of Tokyo. The elevators are fairly standard and could be easily operated by the customers, but the shop prefers to offer the service of having someone hold the door open for you, push the button for your floor, and bow as you exit.

There is one elevator operator who has been performing the same duties since 2004, according to word of mouth. She never stops grinning and showing enthusiasm for her work. How does she find this job enjoyable? She must get bored doing something so monotonous, right?

A closer look reveals that the elevator operator is actually performing a series of movements rather than just pushing buttons. She starts by singing a songlike salutation to the customers before bowing and waving them in. She then moves gracefully to press the elevator button, as if serving a customer a cup of tea like a geisha.

This is what Csikszentmihalyi calls microflow.

We've all started doodling to pass the time when we were bored in a class or at a conference. or whistling as they painted a wall. If we aren't actually being challenged, we become bored and increase the level of complexity to pass the time. Since we all must perform such tasks, our ability to transform them into microflow moments into something we enjoy is essential to our happiness.

Even Bill Gates does the nightly dishes. He claims he enjoys it, that it helps him unwind and clear his mind, and that he makes an effort to get a little better at it every day by adhering to a set of rules or guidelines he has created for himself, such as placing plates first, forks second, and so on.

One of his daily microflows occurs at this time.

One of the most significant physicists of all time, Richard Feynman, also enjoyed doing routine things. Feynman was hired to work on the creation of a computer that could handle parallel processing when he was already well-known in the world by W. Daniel Hillis, one of the founders of the supercomputer manufacturer Thinking Machines. On his first day of employment, he claims Feynman arrived and inquired, "OK, boss, what's my assignment?" They asked him to work on a specific mathematical problem because they didn't have anything else planned. He said, "That sounds like a bunch of baloney—give me something real to do," as soon as he realized they were giving him a pointless task to keep him occupied.

He was then sent to a nearby store to purchase office supplies, and he finished his assignment while grinning. Feynman committed himself to microflowing, such as painting the office walls, when he didn't have a pressing task to complete or needed to clear his mind.

A group of investors said, "You have a Nobel laureate in there painting walls and soldering circuits," after visiting the Thinking Machines offices a few weeks later.

Instant Vacations: Getting There Through Meditation

We can reach the state of flow more quickly by training our minds. One way to strengthen our mental muscles is through meditation.

There are many different kinds of meditation, but they all aim to calm the mind, observe our thoughts and emotions, and focus on one thing.

The fundamental technique entails sitting upright and paying attention to your breath. Anyone can do it, and after just one session, you can already tell a difference. You can calm the onslaught of thoughts and expand your mental horizons by focusing on the air coming in and going out of your nose.

The Archer's Secret

A seventeen-year-old South Korean girl won the gold medal in archery at the 1988 Summer Olympics. When asked how she trained, she said that spending two hours a day in meditation was the most crucial aspect of her preparation.

Meditation is a fantastic remedy for our smartphones and their notifications that are constantly clamoring for our attention if we want to improve our ability to enter a state of flow.

Worrying about doing it "right," achieving complete mental stillness, or attaining "nirvana" is one of the most common errors made by beginners to meditation. Keeping your attention on the journey is the most crucial thing.

Slowing down the "centrifuge" of the mind, even for a brief moment, can make us feel more rested and give us a sense of clarity because the mind is constantly swirling with thoughts, ideas, and emotions.

In fact, one of the things we discover through meditation practice is how to stop worrying about anything that crosses our mind. Even though the thought of murdering our boss might briefly cross our minds, we simply categorize it as a thought and allow it to vanish like a cloud without passing judgment or rejecting it. One expert claims that it is only one of the sixty thousand thoughts that we have each day.

Brain waves in alpha and theta are produced during meditation. These waves can take up to an hour for a beginner to experience, but they usually appear right away for experienced meditators. These tranquilizing brainwaves are the ones that are triggered just before we go to sleep, while we lie in the sun, or just after a hot bath.

Everywhere we go, we all have a spa with us. Anyone can do it with a little practice; all it takes is the knowledge of how to enter.

Humans as Ritualistic Beings

Life is ritualistic by nature. One might contend that humans naturally engage in routines that keep them busy. We've been coerced in some contemporary cultures to abandon our ritualistic lifestyles in favor of a never-ending quest for success. Nevertheless, people have always been busy throughout history. Hunting, cooking, farming, exploring, and raising families were among our daily activities, which were organized as rituals to keep us occupied.

But in an unusual way, rituals are still ingrained in modern Japan's way of life and business procedures. The three major religions in Japan are Confucianism, Buddhism, and Shintoism, all of which place more emphasis on rituals than on inflexible rules.

Process, manners, and the way you approach a task are more crucial when conducting business in Japan than the outcome. This book is not intended to discuss whether this is good or bad for the economy. It is undeniable, however, that finding flow is much simpler in a "ritualistic workplace" than in one where we are constantly stressed out trying to accomplish unclear goals set by our managers.

Rituals provide us with definite guidelines and goals that enable us to achieve a state of flow. The process, the smaller steps along the way to achieving a goal, are provided by rituals, which help us when we are faced with a single large goal and feel lost or overwhelmed by it. When faced with a challenging objective, try to divide it into manageable pieces and then focus on each piece separately.

Use your daily rituals as tools to achieve flow by concentrating on enjoying them. The result won't matter; it will happen naturally. Happiness is found in the action, not the outcome. Remind yourself: "Rituals over goals," as a general rule.

The most successful people are not necessarily the happiest. They are the ones who are in a state of flow for the longest periods of time.

Using Flow To Find Your Ikigai

After reading this chapter, you ought to have a clearer understanding of the activities in your life that put you in flow. Write them all down on a piece of paper, and then consider the following: What characteristics do the things that get you in the zone all share? Why do those activities make you feel in the zone? Do you prefer practicing your favorite activities alone or with others, for instance? Do you find that you flow better when you're physically active than when you're just thinking?

You may discover the ikigai at the core of your life in the responses to these questions. If you don't, then keep looking by learning more about what you enjoy and investing more time in the things that make you feel in the zone. Try new things that are similar to and curious to you but are not on the list of things that make you flow. For instance, if photography puts you in the zone, you could also try painting; you might even prefer it more! If you enjoy snowboarding but have never tried surfing, for example.

Flow is enigmatic. It works similarly to a muscle: the more you exercise it, the more you'll flow and get closer to your ikigai.

CHAPTER 5

MASTERS OF LONGEVITY

Words Of Wisdom From The Longest-Living People In The World

Flow is mysterious. It works similarly to a muscle: the more you exercise it, the more fluidly you move, and the nearer you are to your ikigai. while working on this book, we wanted to hear from the true masters of this art, not just read about the factors that contribute to a long and happy life.

Although the interviews we conducted in Okinawa deserve their own chapter, we have given an overview of a few international champions of longevity's life ideologies in the section that comes before it. Supercentenarians are those who live to be at least 110 years old.

Norris McWhirter, the editor of The Guinness Book of World Records, first used the phrase in 1970. Following its appearance in Generations by William Strauss and Neil Howe, it was used more frequently in the 1990s. Only about 75 of the estimated 300 to 450 supercentenarians in the world today have had their ages verified. Although they are not superheroes, we may view them as such because they have lived on this planet for a much longer period of time than the average person.

Given the increase in life expectancy across the globe, there may be more supercentenarians. Living a wholesome and meaningful life may enable us to join their ranks.

Let's examine some of what they have to say.

Misao Okawa (117)

"Eat and sleep, and you'll live a long time. You have to learn to relax."

The oldest person still alive as of April 2015, according to the Gerontology Research Group, was Misao Okawa, who passed away in an Osaka, Japan, nursing home after living for 117 years and 27 days.

She was born in 1898, the same year that Spain lost control of its colonies in Cuba and the Philippines, the United States annexed Hawaii, and Pepsi-Cola was first introduced. Her father was a textile merchant. She lived in three different centuries and took care of herself until she was 110.

Misao gave a straightforward response when asked about her self-care routine by professionals: "Eating sushi and sleeping," to which we should add that she has a tremendous thirst for life. She smiled and said,

"I ask myself the same thing," in response to their question about her longevity secret.

Evidence that Japan is still a long-lasting factory: At the age of 112 years and 150 days, Sakari Momoi passed away in July of the same year. He was older than fifty-seven women at the time, but he was the oldest man in the world.

María Capovilla (116)
"I've never eaten meat in my life."

Mara Capovilla, who was born in Ecuador in 1889, holds the record for being the oldest person alive. At 116 years and 347 days old, she passed away from pneumonia in 2006. She was survived by three children, twelve grandchildren, and twenty great- and great-great grandchildren.

At the age of 107, she gave one of her final interviews and shared her thoughts and memories:

I'm grateful to God for keeping me going, and I'm joyful. I had no idea I'd live this long; I had assumed my death years ago. My husband, Antonio Capovilla, was a ship's captain. He died at the age of 84. We had a son and two daughters, and I now have a large number of grandchildren and great-grandchildren.

In earlier times, things were better. People acted more properly. We used to dance, though more subtly; there was one song I especially enjoyed dancing to: "Mara" by Luis Alarcón. I still recall the majority of the words. Additionally, I regularly pray and recall many of them.

I can still dance the waltz, which I like. Additionally, I continue to create crafts and engage in some activities from my student days.

Once her memories of the past were complete, she started dancing, which was one of her great passions, with a vigor that made her appear much younger.

She simply stated, "I don't know what the secret to long life is," in response to the question about her longevity. I don't eat any meat, that's the only thing I do. It is due to that, I believe.

Jeanne Calment (122)
"Everything's fine."

Jeanne Calment, who was born in Arles, France, in February 1875, lived until August 4, 1997, making her, at 122, the oldest person in recorded history. She jokingly claimed that she "competed with Methuselah," and there is no doubt that as she continued to celebrate birthdays, she broke a number of records.

She lived a happy life and almost nothing was taken away from her before she passed away naturally. Even after turning 100, she continued to bicycle. She maintained her independence up until the age of 110, when, following an unintentional small fire in her apartment, she decided to move into a nursing home. When her cataracts made it difficult for her to hold a cigarette to her lips at age 120, she gave up smoking.

Her sense of humor might have been one of her secrets. I see badly, I hear badly, and I feel badly, but everything's fine, she said on her 120th birthday.

Walter Breuning (114)

"If you keep your mind and body busy, you'll be around a long time."

Walter Breuning, who was born in Minnesota in 1896, lived to see three centuries. He had two wives and a fifty-year career on the railroad when he passed away in Montana in 2011 from natural causes. He retired to a Montana assisted living facility at the age of 83 and stayed there until his passing. He is the second-oldest man to have been born in the United States (of verified age).

In his later years, he participated in numerous interviews, adamant that his habit of only eating two meals per day and working for as long as he could were two factors that contributed to his longevity. "Both your body and mind. On his 112th birthday, he declared, "You keep both busy, and you'll be here a long time." He was still working out every day at that time.

Breuning's other secrets included the fact that he frequently assisted others and that he had no fear of passing away. We're all going to die, he said in a 2010 interview with the Associated Press. Some people are afraid of passing away. Never be scared of dying. You were created to die.

He reportedly told a pastor before dying in 2011 that he had made a deal with God: If he wasn't going to get better, it was time to go.

Alexander Imich (111)

"I just haven't died yet."
Alexander Imich, a parapsychologist and chemist who lived in the United States and was born in Poland in 1903, held the record for the oldest

man in the world after his predecessor passed away in 2014. Imich passed away shortly after, in June of that same year, leaving behind a lengthy life full of adventures.

Imich credited his long life to many things, including never drinking alcohol. When he was announced as the oldest man in the world, he said, "It's not like I've won the Nobel Prize. I never imagined I'd live to be so old. He replied, "I don't know, when asked what his secret was to living so long. I've just not passed away yet.

Ikigai Artists

Nevertheless, supercentenarians are not the only ones who know the secret to a long life. There are many elderly individuals who provide us with motivation and suggestions for enhancing the meaning and vitality of our lives, despite the fact that they haven't broken any Guinness World Records.

This power is demonstrated by artists who continue to practice their ikigai rather than giving it up.

All forms of art are ikigai that give our lives joy and meaning. All people can access and enjoy beauty, whether they choose to create it or not.

Hokusai, a Japanese artist who produced ukiyo-e woodblock prints and lived for 88 years between the middle of the eighteenth and the middle of the nineteenth century, added the following postscript to the initial printing of his One Hundred Views of Mount Fuji:

Before I turned 70, nothing I produced was worth counting. At 73 years old, I have made some progress toward understanding the true nature of animals, plants, birds, fish, and insects; as a result, at 80 years old, I will have made even more progress; at 90 years old, I hope to have gained insight into the nature of things; at 100 years old, I should have attained a clearly marvelous degree; and at 110 years old, everything I do—every point and every line—will be instinct with life.

The following pages contain some of the most uplifting quotes from the artists Camille Sweeney of the New York Times interviewed. Nobody can stop you when you have a clear purpose, as evidenced by the fact that none of the survivors have retired and are still actively engaged in their passions, which they intend to do until they pass away.

At the age of 86, actor Christopher Plummer, who is still performing, expresses a sinister wish held by many who adore their line of work: "We want to drop dead onstage. That would be a nice dramatic move to make.

This sentiment was shared by Osamu Tezuka, the creator of contemporary Japanese manga. "Please, just let me work," he pleaded in his final cartoon before passing away in 1989.

On a stroll through Paris, the 86-year-old filmmaker Frederick Wiseman said that he enjoys his work, which is why he puts so much effort into it. Everyone moans about their aches, pains, and other discomforts, but my friends are either gone or still employed, he said.

Carmen Herrera, a painter who has just turned 100, sold her first piece of art when she was eighty-nine years old. The Tate Modern and the Museum of Modern Art currently have her pieces in their permanent collections. She stated, "I am always waiting to finish the next thing," in response to a question about how she saw her future. absurd, I realize. I progress every day.

"You may grow old and trembling in your anatomies, you may lie awake at night listening to the disorder of your veins, you may miss your only love, you may see the world about you devastated by evil lunatics, or know your honour trampled in the sewers of baser minds. There is only one thing for it then—to learn. Learn why the world wags and what wags it. That is the only thing which the mind can never exhaust, never alienate, never be tortured by, never fear or distrust, and never dream of regretting."

—*T. H. White*, **The Once and Future King**

Edward O. Wilson, a writer and naturalist, remarked, "I feel I have enough experience to join those who are addressing big questions. I was shocked at how little this was being done when I started reading and thinking more broadly about the questions of what we are, where we came from, and where we are going about ten years ago.

The idea that we lose our mental faculties as we get older is, in part, a myth, according to Ellsworth Kelly, an artist who passed away in 2015 at the age of 92. Instead, he claimed that as we age, we gain more clarity and the ability to observe more clearly. One advantage of growing older is that you gain more knowledge. I still discover new things every day. Thus, fresh paintings are present.

The architect Frank Gehry, who is now 86 years old, reminds us that it can take seven years to complete some buildings "from the time you're hired until you're finished,"14 a fact that encourages patience with the passage of time. But the man in charge of the Guggenheim Museum in Bilbao is adept at staying in the present: "You stay in your time. You never turn around. I believe that if you relate to the time you're in, keep your eyes and ears open, read the news, stay interested in everything, and keep your curiosity alive, you will naturally be in your time.

Longevity in Japan

Although there are many centenarians living in isolated villages abroad, many of those verified as having lived the longest are found in the United States due to its extensive civil registry. People who have lived through a century seem to live fairly typical lives in the country.

Japan has the highest life expectancy of any nation in the world, making it the global superstar of longevity. Longevity in Japan is closely linked to its culture, as we will see later, in addition to a healthy diet, which we will discuss in detail, and an integrated health care system in which people visit the doctor for routine checkups to prevent disease.

The Japanese have a strong sense of community and strive to remain active right up until the end, which is a big part of their longevity secret.

There must be an ikigai on your horizon, a goal that directs your life and motivates you to create things of beauty and utility for the community and yourself, if you want to keep busy even when there is no need to work.

CHAPTER 6

LESSONS FROM JAPAN'S CENTENARIANS

Traditions And Proverbs For Happiness And Longevity

We had to take a nearly three-hour flight from Tokyo to Naha, Okinawa's capital, in order to get to Ogimi. We had informed the Village of Longevity's town council of our plans to visit the area and conduct interviews with the locals who were the oldest several months prior. We eventually received the support we needed after several conversations and were able to rent a home just outside the town

We discovered ourselves at the doorstep of some of the world's longest-living individuals a year after we began this project.

We noticed right away that it appeared as though time had stopped there and everyone in the town was existing in the present moment without end.

Arriving In Ogimi

We are able to stop worrying about the traffic after two hours of driving from Naha. We have the ocean and a deserted beach to our left and the mountainous Yanbaru forests of Okinawa to our right.

Route 58 skirts the coast until it reaches Ogimi after passing Nago, the home of Okinawa's famed Orion beer. In the small area of land between the road and the mountain's base, a few tiny homes and shops will sporadically appear.

As we enter the municipality of Ogimi, we pass a few small groups of houses strewn about, but the town doesn't really seem to have a center. We eventually arrive at the Center for the Support and Promotion of Well-Being, which is housed in an unattractive cinderblock structure just off the highway, thanks to our GPS.

We enter through the back door, and Taira, a man, is there to greet us. A small, vivacious woman introducing herself as Yuki is standing next to him. Immediately, two more women get up from their desks and direct us to a conference room. They offer us each a cup of green tea and a few shikuwasa, a diminutive citrus fruit that, as we will see later, is incredibly nutrient-dense.

Taira, dressed in a suit, takes a seat across from us and unfolds a three-ring binder and a sizable planner. He is seated next to Yuki. A list of every person living in the town is kept in the binder, arranged by age and "club," or moai. Taira emphasizes that Ogimi is known for its communities of people who support one another. The moai operate more like a family than they are organized around any specific goal. Taira also reveals that most activities in Ogimi are motivated by volunteer work rather than financial gain. Everyone offers to help, and the local government handles task delegation. Everyone can feel useful and a part of the community in this way.

Before Cape Hedo, the northernmost point of the largest island in the archipelago, Ogimi is the last town before that.

We can see the entire town below from the peak of one of Ogimi's mountains. We wonder where the nearly 32 hundred residents are hiding because almost everything is the shade of green of the Yanbaru jungle. A few houses are visible, but they are dispersed and located in small valleys or close to the sea, both of which are reached by side roads.

Communal life

The only three tables in one of Ogimi's few restaurants are already reserved when we arrive, despite our invitation to eat there.

We'll head to Churaumi instead, so don't worry. Yuki says as she makes her way back to her car, "It never fills up.

She takes great pride in the fact that she is still driving at the age of 88. Ninety-nine-year-old copilot has also chosen to spend the day with us. We have to travel quickly on a highway that occasionally has more dirt than asphalt to keep up with them. We can finally eat once we make it to the other side of the jungle.

Yuki says as we take our seats, "I don't really go to restaurants. Nearly all of my food comes from my vegetable garden, and Tanaka, a longtime friend, is where I get my fish from.

The eatery is close to the water and resembles something from the Star Wars planet Tatooine. The "slow food" prepared with locally grown organic vegetables is boasted about on the menu in big letters.

However, food is actually not that important, says Yuki. She is extroverted and quite attractive. She enjoys discussing her position as the director of several associations that are run by the local government.

She offers a bite of the tiny confection that came after our meal, saying, "Food won't help you live longer." "Smiling and having fun are the keys,"

Ogimi has only a few eateries and no bars, but its residents lead active social lives centered around their local community centers. The town is divided into seventeen distinct neighborhoods, each of which is led by a president and has a number of administrators in charge of things like culture, celebrations, social activities, and longevity.

This final category receives close attention from the locals.

One of the seventeen neighborhoods has extended an invitation to us to their community center. It is a dilapidated structure next to a mountain in the Yanbaru jungle, which is home to the town's famous sprites, the bunagaya.

The Bunagaya Spirits Of The Yanbaru Jungle

Magical beings known as bunagaya live close to Ogimi and the towns nearby in the Yanbaru jungle. They appear as children with long red hair who enjoy hiding in gajumaru (banyan) trees in the jungle and going beach fishing.

Bunagaya sprites appear in a lot of the myths and legends of Okinawa. They are unpredictable, naughty, and playful. It is believed by the locals that if you want to make friends with the bunagaya, you must respect nature. They are said to love the mountains, rivers, sea, trees, earth, wind, and animals.

A BIRTHDAY PARTY

We are welcomed by a group of about twenty people when we enter the neighborhood's community center. They proudly announce, "The youngest among us is eighty-three!"

We sit around a big table and have our interviews while sipping green tea. After we're done, we're taken to a venue where we celebrate three of the group members' birthdays. One "young man" has just turned eighty-nine, one woman is turning ninety-nine, another is turning ninety-four.

We end with an English rendition of "Happy Birthday" after singing a few of the village's most well-known songs. blows out the candles and expresses gratitude to everyone for attending her party as she celebrates turning 99. We eat homemade shikuwasa cake and end up dancing and having a party as though it were a twentysomething's birthday.

Although it's the first party we'll go to during our week in the village, it won't be the last. A traditional festival with local bands, dancers, and food stands will be held at the base of a mountain, and we'll also participate in karaoke with some seniors who can sing better than we can.

Celebrate Each Day, Together

In Ogimi, celebrations seem to be an integral part of daily life.

Gateball is one of the most well-liked sports among older Okinawans, and we're invited to watch a game. It entails using a stick resembling a mallet to strike a ball. It is a low-impact sport that can be played anywhere and is a great reason to get moving and have a good time with your friends. There is no upper age limit for contestants in the neighborhood competitions.

In the weekly game, we compete and fall short to a woman who just turned 104. Everyone applauds, and the defeated expression on our faces makes people laugh.

The residents of the village must practice spirituality in order to be happy, in addition to playing together and having celebrations as a group.

The gods of Okinawa

Ryukyu Shinto is the predominant religion in Okinawa. Shinto is a language that means "the path of the gods," and Ryukyu was the original name of the Okinawa archipelago. Ryukyu Shinto incorporates shamanism and animism along with elements of Chinese Taoism, Confucianism, Buddhism, and Shintoism.

This ancient belief holds that there are countless spirits inhabiting the world, which are further subdivided into spirits of the house, the forest, the trees, and the mountains. Through festivals and rituals, as well as by dedicating sacred spaces, it is crucial to appease these spirits.

A large number of the two main types of temples—the utaki and the uganju—can be found in Okinawa's sacred jungles and forests. Next to a waterfall in Ogimi, we went to an uganju, or little open-air temple, which was decorated with incense and coins. People go to the utaki, a group of stones, to pray and, according to legend, to commune with the afterlife.

While traditional Shintoism is true in the rest of Japan, women are regarded as having a higher spiritual status than men in Okinawa's religious practice. Yuta are females who have been selected by their communities to serve as their mediums, allowing them to communicate with spirits through customary rituals.

Another significant aspect of spiritual practice in Okinawa and Japan overall is ancestor worship. A butsudan, or small altar, is typically found in the home of the firstborn of each generation, where prayers and offerings are made to the family's ancestors.

Mabui

Every individual possesses a mabui, or essence. Our life force and spirit originate from this mabui. It creates who we are and is eternal.

Sometimes the mabui of the dead is imprisoned in the body of the living. When a person dies suddenly, especially at a young age, and his or her mabui refuses to enter the afterlife, this situation necessitates a separation ritual to release the mabui of the deceased.

Physical contact is another method of transmitting a mabui. A grandmother transfers some of her mabui to her granddaughter when she leaves her a ring. Photographs can also be used as a means of interpersonal communication.

The Older, the Stronger

Looking back, we can say that our days in Ogimi were both intense and carefree, much like the way of life of the locals, who at first glance always seemed to be busy with important tasks but who, upon closer inspection, did everything with a sense of calm. They were never hurried, even though they were constantly pursuing their ikigai.

They appeared to be happily engaged in their work, but we also observed that they adhered to the other guidelines for happiness put forth by Washington Burnap 200 years ago: "The grand essentials to happiness in this life are something to do, something to love, and something to hope for."

We went to a small market on the outskirts of town on our final day to purchase gifts. Only locally grown produce, green tea, shikuwasa juice, and water bottles labeled "Longevity Water" from a spring tucked away in the Yanbaru forests are offered for sale there.

We bought some of this Longevity Water for ourselves and sipped it while sitting in the parking lot and gazing at the water, hoping that the tiny bottles that contained a magical elixir would grant us health, long lives, and aid us in discovering our own ikigai. Then we posed for a picture next to a bunagaya statue and approached it one last time to read the inscription:

A Declaration from the Town Where People Live Longest

At 80 I am still a child.
When I come to see you at 90,
send me away to wait until I'm 100.
The older, the stronger;
let us not depend too much on our children as we age.
If you seek long life and health, you are welcome in our
   village,
where you will be blessed by nature,
and together we will discover the secret to longevity.
April 23, 1993
Ogimi Federation of Senior Citizen Clubs

The Interviews

We interviewed the oldest residents of the community 100 times over the course of a week, asking them about their life philosophy, ikigai, and the keys to longevity. For a short documentary, we used two cameras to record these conversations, and we selected a few particularly poignant and uplifting quotes to use in this chapter of the book.

Don't worry

"Not worrying is the key to living a long life. Don't let your heart age; instead, keep it young. With a pleasant smile on your face, open your heart to others. Everyone will want to see you if you smile and are open in your heart, including your grandchildren.

Going outside and introducing yourself to people is the best way to prevent anxiety. Every day I do it. I go there and greet people and say, "Hello!"

and "See you later!" After that, I tend to my vegetable garden at home. I socialize with my friends in the afternoon.

People get along well here. To avoid creating issues, we strive. The only thing that matters is having fun and spending time with each other.

Cultivate good habits

"Every morning when I open the curtains to see my garden, where I grow my own vegetables, I feel joy. I immediately go outside to inspect my tomatoes, mandarin oranges, and other produce. The sight of them calms me, and I adore it. I spend an hour in the garden before returning inside to prepare breakfast.

"My own vegetables are grown, and I prepare them myself. Ikigai for me is that.

"Your fingers hold the key to maintaining mental acuity as you age. back and forth from your fingers to your brain. You can live to be 100 if you keep your fingers busy.

"I get up at four every day. I set my alarm for that time, have a cup of coffee, and do a little exercise, lifting my arms. That gives me energy for the rest of the day."

"I eat a bit of everything; I think that's the secret. I like variety in what I eat; I think it tastes better."

"Working. If you don't work, your body breaks down."

"When I wake up, I go to the *butsudan* and light incense. You have to keep your ancestors in mind. It's the first thing I do every morning."

"I wake up every day at the same time, early, and spend the morning in my vegetable garden. I go dancing with my friends once a week."

"I do exercise every day, and every morning I go for a little walk."

"I never forget to do my taiso exercises when I get up."

"Eating vegetables—it helps you live longer."

"To live a long time you need to do three things: exercise to stay healthy, eat well, and spend time with people."

Nurture your friendships every day

"My favorite ikigai is hanging out with my friends. It's crucial that we all gather here and talk. It's one of my favorite things in life to know that I'll see them all again tomorrow.

"Hanging out with friends and neighbors is my main hobby."

"The key to a long life is talking to the people you love every day," someone once said.

"I wave at everyone who drives by me and say hello and "See you later" to the kids on their way to school. Drive carefully, I exhort. I'm outside on my feet the entire time between 7:20 and 8:15 a.m., greeting people. When everyone has left, I return inside.

"Chatting and drinking tea with my neighbors. That's the best thing in life. And singing together."

"I wake up at five every morning, leave the house, and walk to the sea. Then I go to a friend's house and we have tea together. That's the secret to long life: getting together with people, and going from place to place."

Live an unhurried life

"My secret to living a long life is telling myself to slow down and relax all the time. If you're not rushed, you live longer.

"I create items out of wicker. My ikigai is that. I always pray right after I wake up. I work out after that and eat breakfast. I calmly get to work on my wicker at seven. I go see my friends when I get tired at five.

"Working on a variety of projects every day. Maintaining constant activity while focusing on one task at a time to avoid becoming overloaded

"The secret to long life is going to bed early, waking up early, and going for a walk. Living peacefully and enjoying the little things. Getting along with your friends. Spring, summer, fall, winter... enjoying each season, happily."

Be optimistic

"I promise myself every day that today will be full of health and energy. Live each moment to the fullest."

"Despite being 98 years old, I still feel young. There is still so much to do.

"Laugh. The most important thing is to laugh. I smile everywhere I go.

"I'll live to be a hundred years old. I'm sure I am! This greatly inspires me. "The best thing in life is dancing and singing with your grandchildren." "I consider myself very lucky to have been born here. I am grateful for it every day.

"Keeping a smile on your face is the most important thing in Ogimi, in life."

"I do volunteer work to give back to the village a bit of what it has given to me. For example, I use my car to help friends get to the hospital."

"There's no secret to it. The trick is just to live."

Keys to the Ogimi Lifestyle

- Every single person we spoke with has a vegetable garden, and the majority of them also have fields of tea, mangoes, shikuwasa, and other crops.
- All of them are a part of a neighborhood organization, where they experience a sense of belonging and support.
- They constantly celebrate, even the little things. Dance, song, and music are integral components of daily life.
- They serve a significant purpose, or perhaps several, in life. They have an ikigai, but they are not overly serious about it. They are at ease and have fun doing everything.

- They take great pride in their traditions and regional culture.

- Regardless of how insignificant something may seem, they are passionate about everything they do

- Locals are extremely passionate about yuimaaru—recognizing the bond between individuals. They assist one another with everything, from farm work (harvesting sugarcane or planting rice) to home construction and community projects. When we had dinner with him on our final night in town, our friend Miyagi informed us that he was constructing a new house with the assistance of all of his friends and that we were welcome to stay there the following time we visited Ogimi.

- Although they are constantly busy, they keep themselves occupied with activities let that them unwind. We didn't see a single elderly grandfather lazing around on a bench. They constantly come and go, whether it's to play a game of gateball, visit with neighbors, or sing karaoke.

CHAPTER 7

THE *IKIGAI* DIET

What the world's longest-living people eat and drink

Japan has the highest life expectancy in the world, at 85 years for men and 87.3 years for women, according to the World Health Organization. Additionally, it has the highest proportion of centenarians per million people in the entire world, at over 520. (as of September 2016).

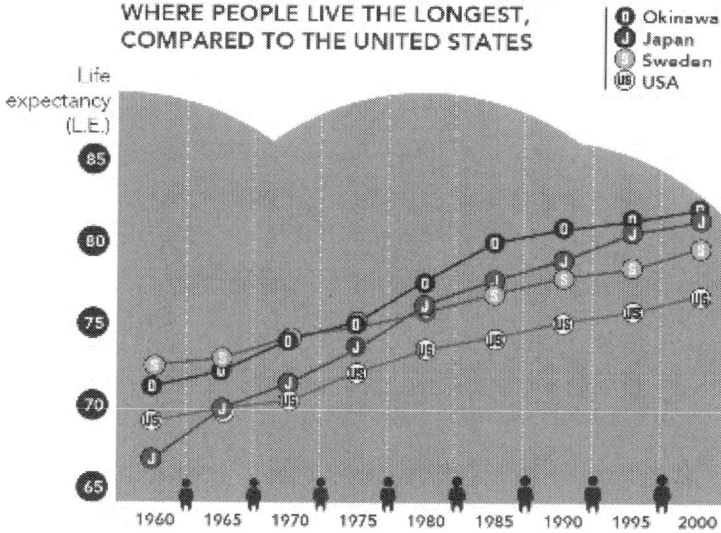

LIFE EXPECTANCY IN THE COUNTRIES
WHERE PEOPLE LIVE THE LONGEST,
COMPARED TO THE UNITED STATES

Legend: Okinawa, Japan, Sweden, USA

Source: World Health Organization, 1966; Japanese Ministry of Health, Labor and Welfare, 2004; U.S. Department of Health and Human Services/CDC, 2005

While life expectancy in Japan is generally high, Okinawa outperforms the country as shown in the above graph comparing life expectancy in Japan, its province Okinawa, Sweden, and the United States.

158

One of the regions of Japan most impacted by World War II was Okinawa. The average life expectancy was not very high in the 1940s and 1950s, not only because of battles on the battlefield, but also because of hunger and a lack of resources after the war. However, as Okinawans rebuilt their lives after the devastation, they became some of the population's longest-living residents.

What longevity secrets do the Japanese possess? What makes Okinawa the best of the best when it comes to life expectancy?

One thing that experts point out is that Okinawa is the only Japanese province without trains. When not driving, its residents must travel by foot or bicycle. Additionally, it is the only province that has been successful in adhering to the government of Japan's advice to consume less than ten grams of salt per day.

Okinawa's miracle diet

Okinawa has the lowest cardiovascular mortality rate in Japan, and diet almost certainly plays a significant role in this. The "Okinawa Diet" is frequently discussed at nutrition panels all over the world, and this is not by accident.

Studies by Makoto Suzuki, a cardiologist at the University of the Ryukyus, who has published more than 700 scientific articles on nutrition and aging in Okinawa since 1970, provide the most specific and frequently cited information on diet in Okinawa.

When they joined Makoto Suzuki's research team, Bradley J. Willcox and D. Craig Willcox wrote The Okinawa Program, which is regarded as the industry standard. They arrived at the subsequent conclusions:

- Locals eat a variety of foods, but vegetables are especially popular. I think the key is variety. Okinawa's centenarians were found to regularly consume 206 different foods, including spices, according to a study of the population. In stark contrast to our fast-food culture's nutritional deficiency, they consumed an average of 18 different foods per day.

- They consume a daily minimum of five servings of fruits and vegetables. Okinawans regularly consume at least seven different kinds of fruits and vegetables. Making sure you're "eating the rainbow" is the simplest way to determine if there is enough variety on your table. For instance, a plate with red peppers, carrots, spinach, cauliflower, and eggplant offers a lot of color and variety. The foundation of an Okinawan's diet is produce, including vegetables, potatoes, legumes, and soy products like tofu. Vegetables account for more than 30% of their daily caloric intake.

- The staple food of their diet is grain. Every day, white rice is consumed by the Japanese, occasionally with noodles. The staple food in Okinawa is also rice.

- They eat sugar infrequently and only cane sugar when they do. Every morning on the way to Ogimi, we passed through a number of sugarcane fields. At Nakijin Castle, we even sipped a glass of cane juice. There was a sign describing sugarcane's anticarcinogenic properties next to the booth selling the juice.

In addition to these fundamental nutritional guidelines, Okinawans consume fish three times on average per week, unlike in other regions of Japan where pork is more commonly consumed, though only once or twice per week by locals.

In this regard, Makoto Suzuki's research suggests that:

- Okinawans generally consume one-third less sugar than the rest of Japan's population, which means that they eat far fewer desserts and chocolate.

- In addition, they consume less salt than the rest of Japan: 7 grams per day as opposed to an average of 12.
- Compared to the rest of Japan, they consume fewer calories: 1,785 on average per day as opposed to 2,068. In fact, the five Blue Zones all have low calorie intake.

Hara hachi bu

This brings up the 80 percent rule, or hara hachi bu in Japanese, that we mentioned in the first chapter. It's simple: Just stop eating when you realize you're almost full but could still eat a little more.

Skipping dessert is a simple way to start putting the idea of hara hachi bu into practice. alternatively, to make portions smaller. The goal is to finish with a slight appetite remaining.

Because of this, portions are frequently much smaller in Japan than in the West. There are no separate appetizers, entrées, and dessert courses. Instead, it's much more typical to see everything served on small plates all at once, including a bowl of miso soup, a plate of vegetables, rice, and something to snack on. In addition to facilitating the varied diet discussed at the beginning of this chapter, serving food on numerous small plates makes it simpler to avoid eating too much.

Hara hachi bu is a long-established custom. Zazen Youjinki, a book on Zen Buddhism written in the twelfth century, advises eating two-thirds of what you might want to. All Buddhist temples in the East practice eating less than one might want. Maybe Buddhism understood the advantages of calorie restriction more than nine centuries ago.

So, Eat Less To Live Longer?

Few would disagree with this notion. Eating fewer calories than our bodies require seems to lengthen life, obviously without going to the extreme of malnutrition. Eating foods with high nutritional value, particularly "superfoods," and staying away from those that increase our overall calorie intake but provide little to no nutritional benefit are the keys to staying healthy while consuming fewer calories.

The calorie restriction we've been talking about is one of the best ways to lengthen your life. When the body regularly consumes enough, or too many, calories, it becomes lethargic and begins to wear out, using a lot of energy just for digestion.

The reduction of IGF-1 (insulin-like growth factor 1) levels in the body is another advantage of calorie restriction. An abundance of the protein IGF-1 in the blood appears to be one of the factors that contribute to the aging process in both humans and animals.

Though it is still unknown if caloric restriction will lengthen human lifespan, mounting evidence suggests that moderate caloric restriction combined with adequate nutrition has powerful protective effects against obesity, type 2 diabetes, inflammation, hypertension, and cardiovascular disease, as well as lowering metabolic risk factors linked to cancer.

Fasting for one or two days a week can be a substitute for adhering to the 80/20 rule every day. The 5:2 diet, also known as the fasting diet, advises consuming no more than 500 calories on two of the seven days of the week while eating normally on the other three.

Fasting has many advantages, including allowing the digestive system to rest and cleaning it.

15 natural antioxidants found in the Okinawan diet

Antioxidants are substances that prevent free radicals from causing harm and hastening the aging process by slowing the oxidation process in cells. For instance, the antioxidant properties of green tea are well known and will be covered in more detail later.

These fifteen foods are regarded as the keys to Okinawan vitality because they are abundant in antioxidants and consumed almost daily in the area:

- Tofu
- Miso
- Tuna
- Carrots
- Goya (bitter melon)
- Kombu (sea kelp)
- Cabbage
- Nori (seaweed)

- Onion

- Soy sprouts

- Hechima (cucumber-like gourd)

- Soybeans (boiled or raw)

- Sweet potato

- Peppers

- Sanpin-cha (jasmine tea)

Sanpin-Cha: The Reigning Infusion In Okinawa

Sanpin-cha, a blend of green tea and jasmine flowers, is the type of tea that Okinawans consume the most of. The jasmine tea that typically originates from China would be the closest equivalent in the West. The Okinawa Institute of Science and Technology's Hiroko Sho conducted a study in 1988 that found jasmine tea lowers blood cholesterol levels.

In Okinawa, sanpin-cha is available in a wide variety of forms, including vending machines. It boasts the advantages of jasmine in addition to all the antioxidant advantages of green tea, which include:

- Reducing the risk of heart attack
- Strengthening the immune system
- Helping relieve stress
- Lowering cholesterol

Okinawans consume three cups of Sanpin-cha on average each day. Even though it might be challenging to locate the exact same blend in the West, we can still enjoy a cup of green tea or even jasmine tea.

The Secrets Of Green Tea

For many years, green tea has been thought to have important medicinal properties. Recent studies have attested to the importance of this ancient plant in the longevity of those who drink it frequently and have confirmed its many advantages.

Green tea originated in China and has only recently spread to the rest of the world, despite being consumed there for millennia. It is air-dried without fermentation, unlike other teas, so it retains its active ingredients even after being dried and crumbled. It provides significant health advantages like:

- Controlling cholesterol
- Lowering blood sugar levels
- Improving circulation
- Protection against the flu (vitamin C)
- Promoting bone health (fluoride)
- Protection against certain bacterial infections
- Protection against UV damage
- Cleansing and diuretic effects

White tea may be even more effective against aging due to its high polyphenol content. In fact, one cup of white tea may have the same antioxidant impact as about a dozen glasses of orange juice, making it the natural product with the highest antioxidant power in the world.

In conclusion, consuming green or white tea regularly can help us maintain a youthful appearance by lowering the levels of free radicals in our bodies.

The powerful *shikuwasa*

The citrus fruit that best represents Okinawa is shikuwasa, and Ogimi is the country's top supplier of it.

Due to the fruit's extreme acidity, shikuwasa juice must be diluted with water before consumption. It has a flavor that falls somewhere between that of a lime and a mandarin orange, to which it is related.

Shikuwasas also contain a lot of nobiletin, an antioxidant-rich flavonoid.

Nobiletin content is high in all citrus fruits, including grapefruits, oranges, and lemons, but shikuwasas from Okinawa have forty times as much as oranges do. It has been demonstrated that ingesting nobiletin can help us avoid developing arteriosclerosis, cancer, type 2 diabetes, and obesity in general.

Hikuwasas also contain minerals, beta carotene, and vitamins C and B1. They are squeezed to make juice and are used in many traditional dishes to flavor food. We were served shikuwasa cake while conducting research at the birthday celebrations of the town's "grandparents."

The Antioxidant Canon, For Westerners

In 2010 the UK's *Daily Mirror* published a list of foods recommended by experts to combat aging. Among these foods readily available in the West are:

- Vegetables such as broccoli and chard, for their high concentration of water, minerals, and fiber
- Oily fish such as salmon, mackerel, tuna, and sardines, for all the antioxidants in their fat
- Fruits such as citrus, strawberries, and apricots; they are an excellent source of vitamins and help eliminate toxins from the body
- Berries such as blueberries and goji berries; they are rich in phytochemical antioxidants
- Dried fruits, which contain vitamins and antioxidants, and give you energy
- Grains such as oats and wheat, which give you energy and contain minerals
- Olive oil, for its antioxidant effects that show in your skin
- Red wine, in moderation, for its antioxidant and vasodilatory properties
- Refined sugar, grains, prepared foods, processed baked goods, and cow's milk and all of its byproducts should all be avoided. You will feel younger and the process of premature aging will be slowed if you follow this diet.

CHAPTER 8

GENTLE MOVEMENTS, LONGER LIFE

Exercises from the East that promote health and longevity Studies from the Blue Zones show that people who move more than others tend to live longer than those who exercise the most

We learned that even those who are over eighty and ninety are still very active when we traveled to Ogimi, the Village of Longevity. They don't just sit around the house reading the newspaper and staring out the window. Residents of Ogimi get up early, go for long walks, sing karaoke with their neighbors, and weed their gardens as soon as breakfast is finished, if not earlier. They don't go to the gym or work out very hard, but they practically never stop moving throughout their daily activities.

As Easy as Getting out of Your Chair

"Metabolism decreases by 90% after 30 minutes of sitting. The enzymes slow down, allowing the bad fat to take longer to travel from your arteries to your muscles, where it can be burned off. And after two hours, the good cholesterol decreases by 20%. Things will start moving again after only five minutes of standing up. Gavin Bradley[1] says in a 2015 interview with Brigid Schulte for the Washington Post that "these things are so basic they're almost stupid." [2] One of the foremost authorities on the subject, Bradley also serves as the director of a global group that promotes health awareness about the dangers of constant sitting.

Living in a city may make it difficult for us to engage in regular, healthy movement, but we can still benefit from exercises that have been shown to be beneficial to the body for hundreds of years.

Although the Eastern practices for achieving balance of the body, mind, and soul have gained a lot of popularity in the West, they have been practiced for centuries in their home nations to support health.

Among other practices, qigong, tai chi, and yoga, which originated in India but is hugely popular in Japan, aim to harmonize the body and mind so that practitioners can face the outside world with courage, joy, and serenity.

The claim that they are elixirs of youth has been supported by science.

These gentle exercises are ideal for older people who have a harder time maintaining their fitness and offer exceptional health benefits.

Tai chi has been demonstrated to improve circulation, muscle tone, and flexibility, as well as to slow the progression of Parkinson's disease and osteoporosis. Equally significant are its emotional advantages, such as its excellent defense against stress and depression.

You don't need to run marathons or spend an hour each day in the gym. All you need, as Japanese centenarians demonstrate, is to include movement in your daily routine. One excellent way to do this is to regularly practice one of these Eastern disciplines. The fact that each discipline has clearly defined steps is an added bonus because, as we saw in chapter IV, disciplines with clear rules encourage flow. Feel free to pick a practice that you love and that gets you moving if you don't like any of these specialties.

The practices that encourage health and longevity will be discussed in more detail in the pages that follow, but first, a small taster: a uniquely Japanese morning routine.

Radio taiso

It has been customary to warm up in the morning since before World War II. The "radio" in its name refers to the time when each exercise's instructions were broadcast over the radio, but nowadays people typically perform these movements while watching a television program or an online video that demonstrates the steps.

Promoting a sense of unity among participants is one of the main goals of radio taiso. The exercises are always carried out in groups, typically before the start of the school day or the start of the workday in businesses.

Radio taiso is a morning ritual practiced by 30% of Japanese people, according to statistics, but it was a trait shared by almost all of the people we spoke to in Ogimi. Even the residents of the nursing home we visited made time for it every day for at least five minutes, though some of them performed the exercises in wheelchairs. We joined them for their daily practice, and the rest of the day brought us renewed energy.

When these exercises are performed in a group, they are frequently conducted on a sports field or in a sizable reception hall and frequently involve the use of loudspeakers.

Depending on whether you complete all or just some of the exercises, it will either take five or ten minutes. They concentrate on enhancing joint mobility and dynamic stretching. One of the most well-known radio taiso exercises is as simple as raising your arms above your head and circling them back down. It is a method for waking up the body; it is a simple mobility exercise that is low-intensity and concentrates on working out as many joints as possible.

Although it may seem simple, we can go days in the modern world without lifting our arms above our ears. Consider this: whenever we use a computer, a smartphone, or a book, our arms are at our sides. When reaching into a cabinet or closet, one of the few times we raise our hands above our heads, our ancestors raised their hands over their heads constantly when gathering things from trees. We can practice all of the fundamental bodily movements with the aid of radio taiso.

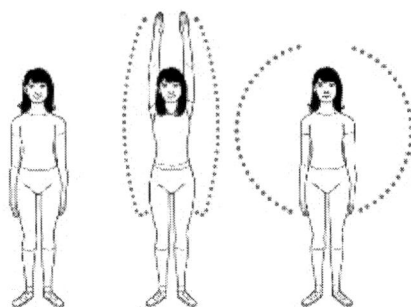

Basic version of the radio taiso exercises (5 minutes).

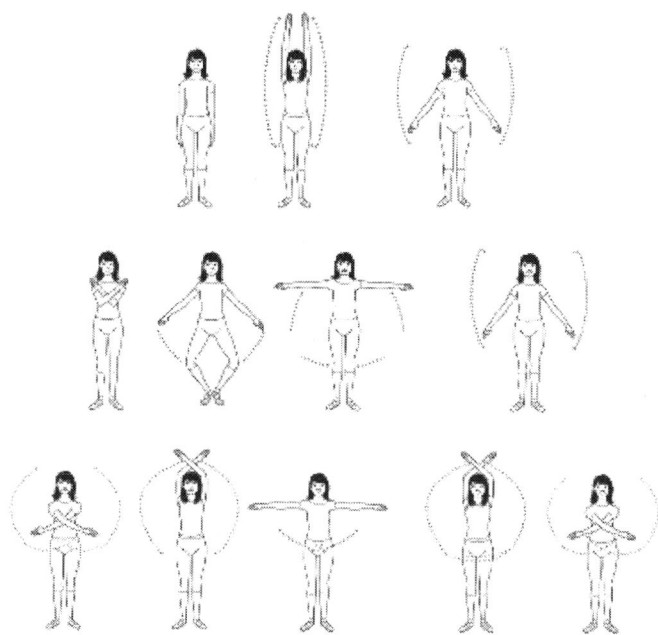

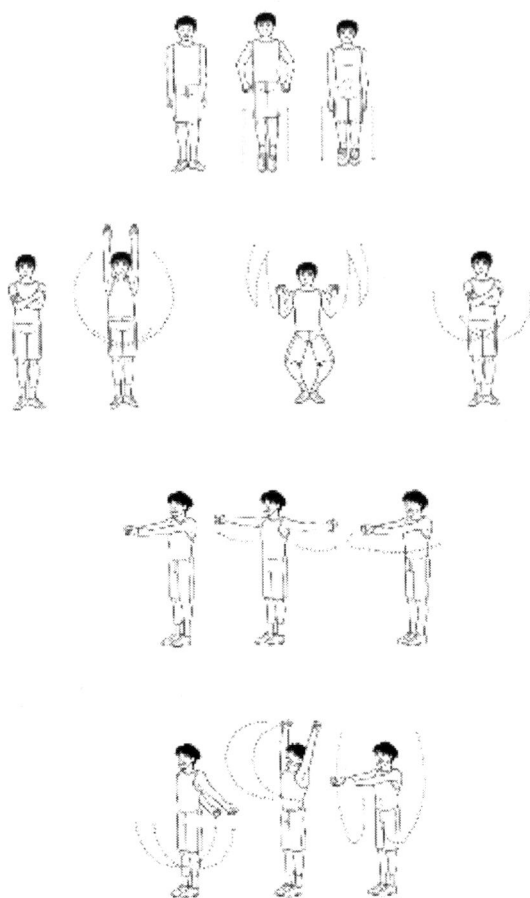

Yoga

Yoga is widely practiced both in the West and Japan and is accessible to almost everyone. Even some of its poses have been modified for practitioners who are expecting or have physical limitations.

Yoga originated in India, where it was created thousands of years ago to connect our mental and physical selves. The term "yoke" in Sanskrit, which refers to the crosspiece that connects draft animals to one another and to the cart they are pulling, is where the word "yoga" originates. Yoga aims to bring the body and the mind into harmony, directing us toward a healthy lifestyle that is in tune with the environment.

The Main Objectives Of Yoga Are:

- To bring us closer to our (human) nature
- Mental and physical purification
- To bring us closer to the divine

Styles Of Yoga

There are many different types of yoga, all of which have similar goals but differ in accordance with the traditions and texts from which they were derived. According to the masters, what separates them is the route taken to reach our highest selves.

Jnana yoga: the yoga of wisdom; the search for discipline and mental growth

Karma yoga: focuses on action, on tasks and duties that benefit oneself and one's community

Bhakti yoga: the yoga of devotion and surrender to the divine

Mantra yoga: focuses on the recitation of mantras to reach a state of relaxation

Kundalini yoga: combines diverse steps to reach the desired mental state

Raja yoga: also known as the royal path; encompasses a range of steps geared toward achieving communion with oneself and others

Hatha yoga: the most widespread form in the West and Japan; characterized by *asanas* or poses combined in a quest for balance

How to do a Sun Salutation

One of the most famous hatha yoga poses is the Sun Salutation. Simply perform the following twelve fundamental movements to accomplish it:

- With your feet together, stand up straight but keep your muscles relaxed. Exhale.
- Take a deep breath in and raise your arms above your head while bending back slightly. Start by placing your hands palms together in front of your chest.
- Exhale as you bend forward until you touch the ground with the palms of your hands, without bending your knees.

- Stretch one leg back to touch the floor with the tips of your toes. Inhale.
- Bring the other leg back, keeping your legs and arms straight, as you hold your breath.
- As you exhale, bend your arms and bring your chest to the ground and then forward, resting your knees on the ground.
- Straighten your arms and bend your spine back, keeping the lower half of your body on the ground. Inhale.
- With your hands and feet on the ground, lift your hips until your arms and legs are straight and your body forms an upside-down V. Exhale throughout the movement.
- The leg you earlier stretched back is brought forward and bent so that your knee and foot are positioned beneath your head and between your hands. Inhale.
- Exhale as you bring your back foot forward and straighten your legs, keeping your hands on the ground as in posture

As you inhale, raise your arms above your head, palms facing inward, and slant your back slightly as you did in posture.

Lower your arms to their initial position in mountain pose while you exhale.

Having just greeted the sun, you are now prepared for an amazing day.

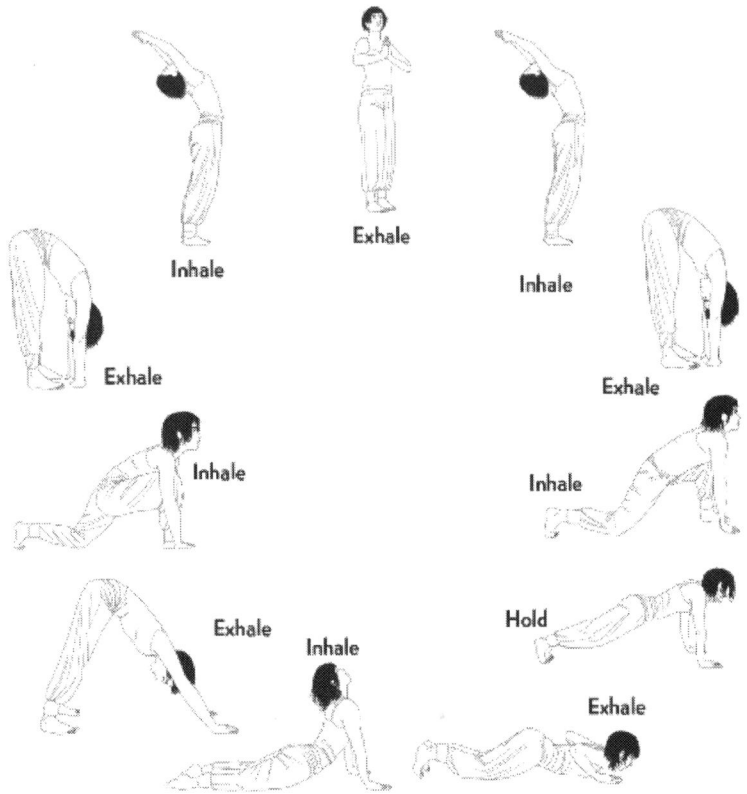

Exhale

Inhale

Inhale

Exhale

Exhale

Inhale

Inhale

Inhale

Hold

Exhale

Exhale

Tai chi

Tai chi, also known as t'ai chi ch'uan (or taijiquan), is a Chinese martial art with roots in Buddhism and Confucianism that has also become very popular in Japan.

189

Zhang Sanfeng, a Taoist master and martial artist, is credited with creating it in Chinese tradition; however, Yang Luchan introduced it to the rest of the world in the nineteenth century.

Tai chi was first a neijia, or internal martial art, with a focus on personal development. With a focus on self-defense, it teaches practitioners how to subdue opponents with the least amount of force and by relying on agility.

Tai chi, which was also thought to be a way of healing the body and the mind, would later be practiced more frequently to promote wellbeing and inner peace. The Chinese government promoted it as an exercise to encourage its people to be more active, so it lost its connection to martial arts and changed to a source of health and well-being that was available to everyone.

Styles of tai chi

There are various tai chi schools and styles. The most well-known are as follows:

Chen-style: alternates between slow movements and explosive ones

Yang-style: the most widespread of the forms; characterized by slow, fluid movements

Wu-style: utilizes small, slow, deliberate movements

Hao-style: centered on internal movements, with almost microscopic external movements; one of the least practiced forms of tai chi, even in China

Despite their differences, these styles all have the same objectives:

1. To control movement through stillness
2. To overcome force through finesse
3. To move second and arrive first
4. To know yourself and your opponent

The ten basic principles of tai chi

The correct application of tai chi is said to adhere to ten fundamental principles, according to master Yang Chengfu:

1. Elevate the crown of your head, and focus all your energy there.
2. Tighten your chest and expand your back to lighten your lower body.
3. Relax your waist and let it guide your body.
4. Learn to differentiate between heaviness and lightness, knowing how your weight is distributed.
5. Relax the shoulders to allow free movement of the arms and promote the flow of energy.
6. Value the agility of the mind over the strength of the body.
7. Unify the upper and lower body so they act in concert.
8. Unify the internal and the external to synchronize mind, body, and breath.

9. Do not break the flow of your movement; maintain fluidity and harmony.

10.   Look for stillness in movement. An active body leads to a calm mind.

Imitating clouds

In the tai chi exercise known as Wave Hands Like Clouds, one of the most popular movements involves mimicking the shape of clouds. These are the actions:

1. Extend your arms in front of you with your palms down.
2. Turn your palms to face in, as though you were hugging a tree trunk.
3. Open your arms out to the side.
4. Bring the left arm up and center, and the right arm down and center.
5. Trace the shape of a ball in front of your body.
6. Turn your left palm toward your face.

7. Shift your weight to your left foot and pivot from your hip toward that side, while your eyes follow the movement of your hand.

8. Bring your left hand to your waist and your right hand in front of your face.

9. Shift your weight to your right foot.

10. Pivot toward your right, looking at your raised right hand the entire time.

11. Repeat this movement fluidly, shifting your weight from one foot to the other as you reposition your hands.

12. Stretch your arms out in front of you again and bring them down slowly, returning to your initial position.

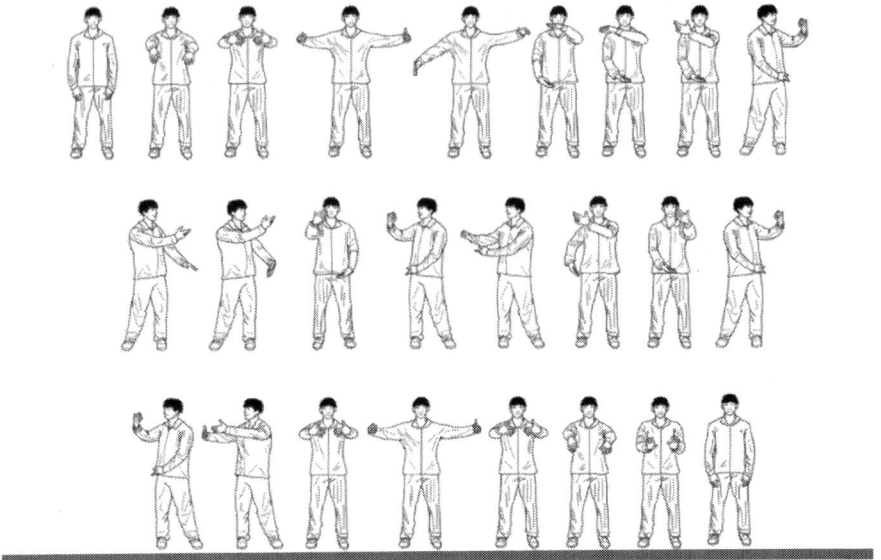

Qigong

Its name, which also goes by the name chi kung, combines the words qi (life force, or energy), and gong (work), denoting that the form utilizes the practitioner's life force. Even though it goes by its current name, the Tao yin, an ancient art meant to promote both physical and mental well-being, is the foundation of qigong, a practice that is relatively modern.

Early in the 20th century, reports on training and martial arts mentioned the technique; by the 1930s, hospitals were using it. Similar to how it had done with tai chi, the Chinese government later made it popular.

Qigong consists of both static and dynamic breathing exercises that can be performed while standing, sitting, or lying down. There are numerous variations of qigong, but they all aim to fortify and regenerate qi. The practice is rigorous despite its typically gentle movements.

Benefits of qigong

Numerous international scientific studies have found that qigong, like tai chi and yoga, has significant health advantages. According to Dr. Kenneth M. Sancier of the San Francisco Qigong Institute, who noted these among those supported by scientific research in his article "Medical Applications of Qigong," the following stand out among them.

- Modification of brain waves
- Improved balance of sex hormones
- Lower mortality rate from heart attacks
- Lower blood pressure in patients with hypertension
- Greater bone density
- Better circulation
- Deceleration of symptoms associated with senility
- Greater balance and efficiency of bodily functions
- Increased blood flow to the brain and greater mind-body connection
- Improved cardiac function
- Reduction in the secondary effects of cancer treatments

By engaging in these arts, we not only stay healthy but also live longer.

Methods for practicing qigong

We must keep in mind that our life energy flows through every part of our body in order to perform qigong properly. We should be able to control its various components.

Tyau Shenn: (regulating the body) by adopting the correct posture—it is important to be firmly rooted to the ground

Tyau Shyi: (regulating the breath) until it is calm, steady, and peaceful

Tyau Hsin: (regulating the mind); the most complicated part, as it implies emptying the mind of thoughts

Tyau Chi: (regulating the life force) through the regulation of the three prior elements, so that it flows naturally

Tyau Shen: (regulating the spirit); the spirit is both strength and root in battle, as Yang Jwing-Ming explains in *The Essence of Taiji Qigong*.

The entire organism will be ready to cooperate in order to accomplish a single goal in this way.

The five elements of qigong

The five elements of earth, water, wood, metal, and fire are represented in a series of qigong exercises that are among the most well-known. This set of exercises aims to harmonize the five energy currents in order to enhance organ and brain function.

These movements can be performed in a variety of ways. In this instance, we're using Professor Mara Isabel Garca Monreal's blueprint from the Barcelona-based Qigong Institute.

EARTH

1. Stand with your legs apart and your feet directly below your shoulders.
2. Turn your feet outward slightly to strengthen the posture.

3. Keep your shoulders relaxed and down and your arms loose at your sides, slightly away from your body (this is the Wu Qi, or rooted, posture).

4. As you inhale, raise your arms in front of you until your hands are level with your shoulders, your palms facing down.

5. Exhale as you bend your knees and bring your arms down until your hands are level with your stomach, your palms facing in.

Hold this position for a few seconds, focusing on your breath.

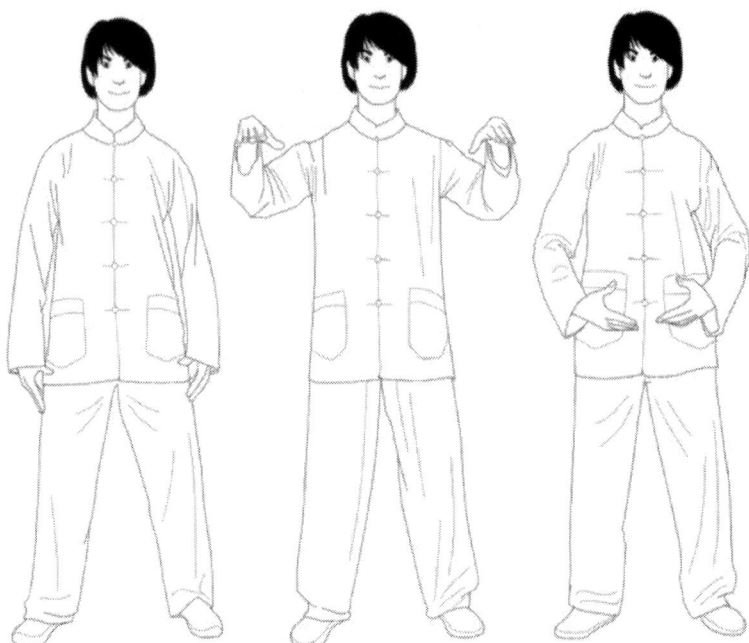

WATER

1. Starting from Earth posture, bend your knees into a squat, keeping your chest upright and exhaling throughout.

2. Press your coccyx downward to stretch your lumbar spine.

3. As you inhale, stand to return to Earth posture.

4. Repeat twice, for a total of three.

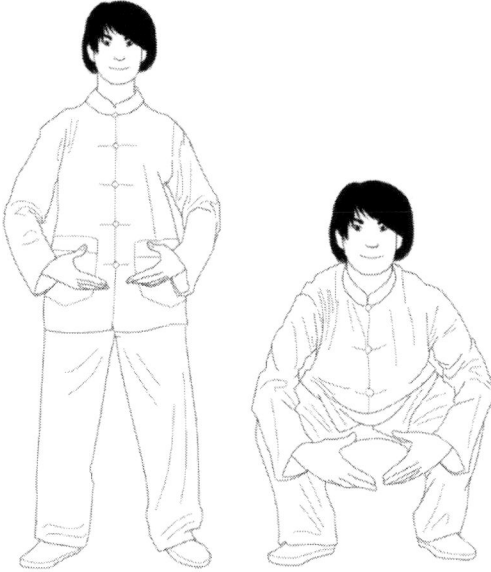

WOOD

- Starting in the Earth position, extend your arms to the side in a circle as you inhale, bringing your hands to a level with your clavicle. At this point, turn your palms upward. Maintaining relaxed shoulders, turn your hands so that the palms and elbows point downward.

- Reverse the movement as you exhale, making a downward circle with your arms until you reach your initial position.

- Repeat twice, for a total of three.

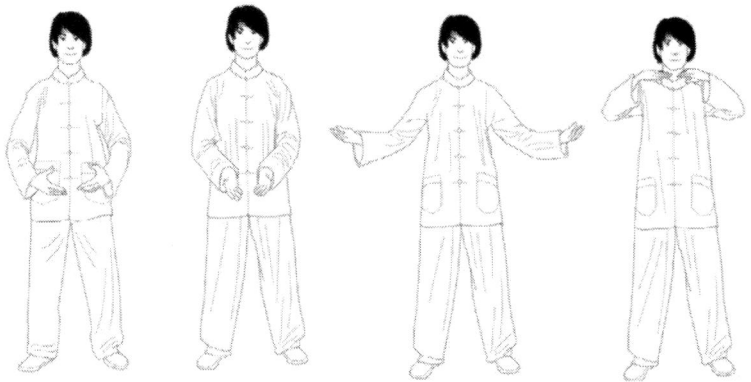

METAL

1. Starting from Earth posture, raise your arms until your hands are level with your sternum.

2. Turn your palms toward each other, about four inches apart, with your fingers relaxed and slightly separated, pointing upward.

3. As you inhale, move your hands away from each other until they are shoulder width apart.

4. As you exhale, bring your hands toward each other until they are back in position .

5. Do this exercise three times, repeating it twice each time. As you bring your hands together in front of your lungs, pay attention to the energy that gathers.

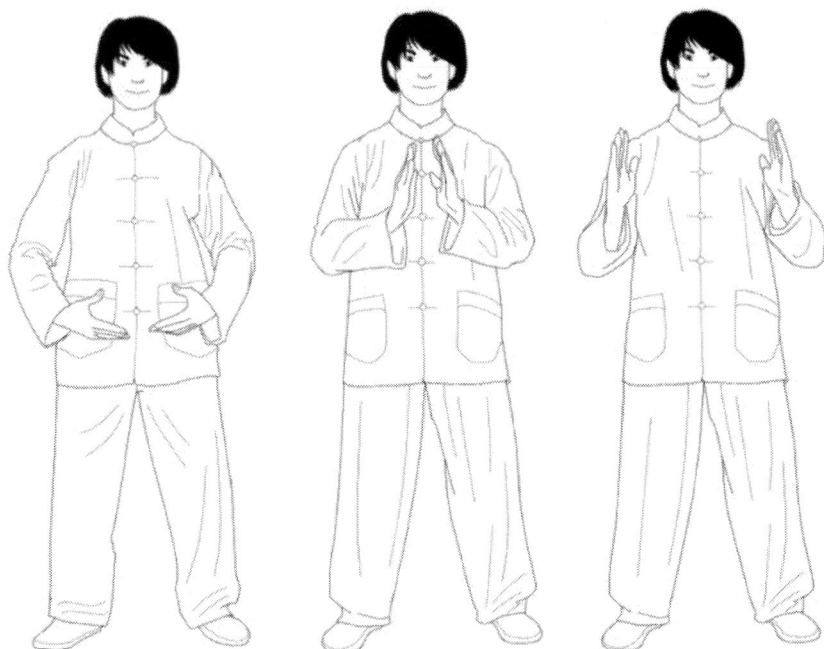

FIRE

1. Starting from Earth posture, bring your hands level with your heart as you inhale, with one hand slightly above the other and your palms facing each other.

2. Rotate your hands to feel the energy of your heart.

3. Turn from your waist gently to the left, keeping your torso relaxed and your forearms parallel to the ground.

4. With your palms still facing each other, separate your hands, bringing one up until it is level with your shoulder, and the other down in front of your abdomen.

5. Turn from your waist gently to the right, keeping your torso relaxed and your forearms parallel to the ground.

6. As you exhale, let your hands come back together in front of your heart.

7. With your palms still facing each other, separate your hands, bringing one up until it is level with your shoulder, and the other down in front of your abdomen.

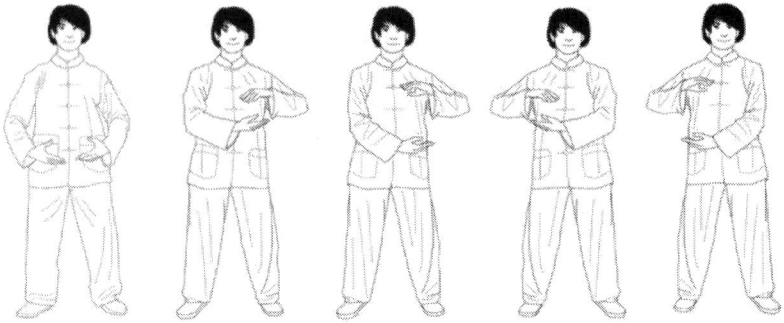

COMPLETING THE SERIES

1. Starting from Earth posture, inhale as you bring your hands level with your shoulders, palms facing down.

2. As you exhale, lower your arms to rest at your sides, returning to the initial Wu Qi posture.

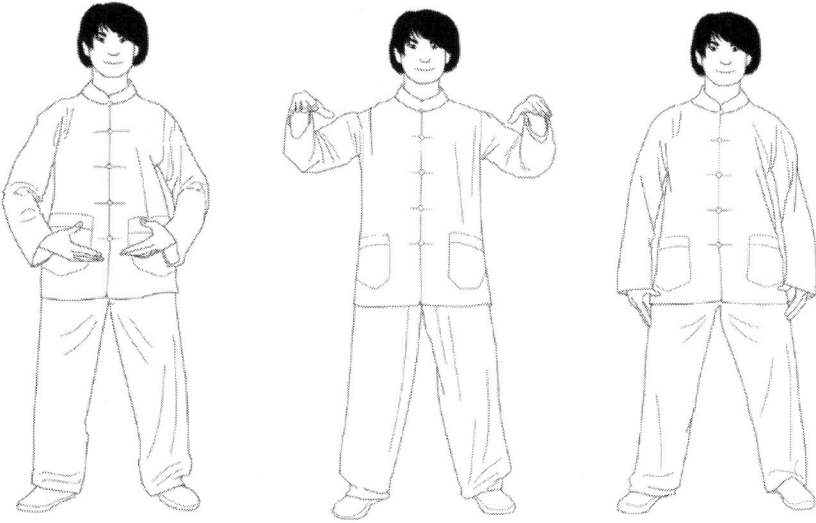

Shiatsu

Shiatsu, which was developed in Japan at the turn of the 20th century primarily to treat arthritis, also stimulates the flow of energy by applying pressure with the thumbs and palms of the hands.

It works to bring the various parts of the body into balance by combining stretching and breathing exercises.

It is not important that a Tao Yin* have a name, is imitating something, or is engraved in jade. What is important is the technique and the essence of what is really practiced. Stretching and contracting, bending and *lifting of the head, stepping, lying down, resting or standing, walking or stepping slowly, screaming or breathing—everything can be a Tao Yin.*

—Ge Hong

Breathe better, live longer

The thirteenth-century text Xiuzhen shishu, also known as Ten Books on the Cultivation of Perfection in the West, is a compilation of information on improving the mind and body from various sources.

It includes quotations from famous Chinese physician and essayist Sun Simiao, who lived in the sixth century, among others. Sun Simiao was an advocate of a method known as the Six Healing Sounds, which involves synchronizing motion, breathing, and sound production with the intention of calming our souls.

The six sounds are:

Xu, pronounced like "shh" with a deep sigh, which is associated with the liver

He, pronounced like "her" with a yawn, which is associated with the heart

Si, pronounced like "sir" with a slow exhale, which is associated with the lungs

Chui, pronounced like "chwee" with a forceful exhale, which is associated with the kidneys

Hoo, pronounced like "who," which is associated with the spleen

Xi, pronounced like "she, " which connects the whole body

Sun Simiao's poem that follows provides guidance on how to live well throughout the season. It emphasizes the value of breathing and advises us to think of the organs connected to each of the therapeutic sounds as we inhale.

In spring, breathe xu for clear eyes and so wood can aid your liver.

In summer, reach for he, so that heart and fire can be at peace.

In fall, breathe si to stabilize and gather metal, keeping the lungs moist.

For the kidneys, next, breathe chui and see your inner waters calm.

The Triple Heater needs your xi to expel all heat and troubles.

In all four seasons, take deep breaths so your spleen can process food.

And, of course, avoid exhaling noisily; don't let even your own ears hear you.

The practice is most excellent and will help preserve your divine elixir.

Being presented with all the Eastern traditions we have discussed in this chapter may feel confusing. The lesson is that they all involve physical activity and breathing awareness. Instead of allowing our mind to be carried away by the sea of daily concerns, these two elements—movement and breath—help us to bring our consciousness in

211

line with our body. We simply aren't conscious of our breathing enough of the time.

CHAPTER 9

RESILIENCE AND *WABI-SABI*

How To Face Life's Challenges Without Letting Stress And Worry Age You

What is resilience?

Everyone with a distinct ikigai pursues their passion regardless of the consequences, which is something that they all have in common. Even when the odds are against them or there are numerous obstacles in their way, they never give up.

We're discussing resilience, which has gained popularity among psychologists.

However, resilience goes beyond the capacity for tenacity. As we'll see in this chapter, it's also a mindset we can develop to keep our attention on what's important in life rather than what is most pressing, as well as to prevent ourselves from becoming overwhelmed by unpleasant feelings.

We'll look at methods for cultivating antifragility in the chapter's final section, which goes beyond resilience.

We all encounter challenging situations sooner or later, and how we handle them can significantly affect our quality of life. To deal with life's ups and downs, proper mental, physical, and emotional resilience training is necessary.

Nana korobi ya oki 七転び八起き

Fall seven times, rise eight.

—Japanese proverb

The capacity to bounce back from setbacks is resilience. We can pick ourselves up and return to what gives our lives purpose more readily the more resilient we are.

People who are resilient know how to maintain their attention on what matters, on their goals, and resist giving in to discouragement. Their adaptability and capacity for change enable them to cope with setbacks and change in fortune. Instead of worrying about the things they cannot control, they focus on the things they can.

Reinhold Niebuhr's well-known Serenity Prayer, in his own words:

God, give us grace to accept with serenity

the things that cannot be changed,

Courage to change the things

which should be changed,

and the Wisdom to distinguish

the one from the other.

Emotional resilience through Buddhism and Stoicism

Siddhartha Gautama (Buddha) was raised in a palace amidst wealth as a prince of Kapilavastu, Nepal. He married and had a child when he was sixteen.

At age 29, he decided to try a different way of life after becoming dissatisfied with his family's wealth and fled the palace to live as an ascetic. But he wasn't looking for asceticism because it didn't bring him the happiness and contentment he needed. Riches or extreme asceticism didn't suit him. He understood that a wise person would not overlook the pleasures of life. While a wise person can tolerate these pleasures, they should always be aware of how simple it is to become compulsively addicted to them.

Zeno of Citium started his education among the Cynics. The Cynics also lived austere lives, renunciating all earthly comforts. The only possessions they had were the clothes on their backs and they lived in the street.

Zeno left the teachings of cynicism after realizing that they did not make him feel happy and founded the school of stoicism, which is based on the principle that there is nothing wrong with enjoying life's pleasures as long as you do not let them rule your life as you do so. Those pleasures will eventually fade, so you must be ready for that.

Instead of eliminating all emotions from our lives, as in cynicism, the purpose is to eradicate negative feelings.

Controlling pleasure, feelings, and desires has been a goal of Buddhism and Stoicism from their inception. Despite having very different philosophies, both work to restrain our egos and negative emotions.

At their core, Buddhism and stoicism are both approaches to cultivating well-being.

Stoicism argues that our pleasures and desires are not the issue. As long as they don't control us, we can enjoy them. Those who could control their emotions were seen as virtues by the Stoics.

What's the worst thing that could happen?

After working hard for a while, we finally land our dream job, but soon we begin looking for something better. We purchase a nice car after winning the lottery, but later decide we need a sailboat in order to survive. When we do manage to win over the person whose heart we've been lusting after, we subsequently discover that our eyes have begun to wander.

It's possible for people to have an insatiable desire.

The Stoics managed to hold that such aspirations and desires are not worth pursuing. Gaining a state of tranquility (apatheia), which is the absence of negative emotions like fear, shame, vanity, and anger and the presence of positive emotions like happiness, love, and serenity, is the goal of virtue

The Stoics engaged in a form of negative visualization, or imagining the worst case scenario in case certain rights and pleasures were taken away from them, in order to maintain their mental virtue.

We must think back on bad things that have happened, but not fret about them, in order to practice negative visualization.

One of the wealthiest men in ancient Rome, Seneca led a luxurious life but was also a practicing Stoic. Every night before going to bed, he advised practicing negative visualization. In fact, he did more than just imagine these bad scenarios; he put them into action, such as by going a week without having servants or the food and drink he was accustomed to as a wealthy man. He was able to respond to the question "What could go wrong?" as a result.

Meditating for healthier emotions

Knowing what we can control and what we can't, as we see in the Serenity Prayer, is another essential element of stoicism, in addition to negative visualization and resisting negative emotions.

Nothing gets accomplished when we worry about things that are out of our control. It will be easier for us to resist giving in to negative emotions if we are clear about what we can change and what we cannot.

Epictetus said, "What matters is how you respond, not what happens to you."

Meditation is a method used in Zen Buddhism to become conscious of our desires and emotions and thus free ourselves from them. The key is to observe our thoughts and emotions as they arise without becoming overwhelmed by them. It is not just a matter of keeping the mind clear of thoughts. By doing this, we can teach our minds to resist feelings of rage, jealousy, or resentment.

"Oṃ maṇi padme hūṃ" is one of the most popular Buddhist mantras, and it focuses on managing negative emotions. O stands for generosity, which purifies the ego, ma stands for ethics, which purifies jealousy, and padme is "h," which is "padme" in Sanskrit. The words is the patience that purifies passion and desire," "pad is the accuracy that purifies bias," "me is the surrender that purifies greed," and "h" are the qualities of wisdom that purify hatred.

The here and now, and the impermanence of things

Knowing when to live is another important aspect of developing resilience. Buddhism and Stoicism both serve as reminders that all there is and all we have control over is the present. We should cherish the present moment and the here and now rather than dwelling on the past or the future.

Thich Nhat Hanh, a Buddhist monk, states that "the only moment in which you can be truly alive is the present moment."

The Stoics advise thinking about how fleeting our surroundings are in addition to living in the moment.

The Roman emperor Marcus Aurelius once said that the things we cherish are similar to a tree's leaves in that they are liable to fall at any time due to a gust of wind. Additionally, he asserted that changes in the environment we live in are not accidental but rather a fundamental aspect of the cosmos, which is actually a Buddhist idea.

Never forget that everything we own and everyone we love will vanish at some point. We ought to keep this in mind, but without succumbing to pessimism. The realization that everything is temporary should inspire us to love the here and now and the people around us rather than making us depressed.

Seneca says that "all things human are transient and brittle."

Every Buddhist discipline is based on the understanding that the world is impermanent, ephemeral, and temporary. This helps us avoid experiencing too much pain when we experience loss.

Wabi-sabi and ichi-go ichi-e

The Japanese idea of wabi-sabi demonstrates the beauty of the transient, changeable, and imperfect nature of the world. We should seek out beauty in imperfect, incomplete things rather than trying to find it in things that are perfect.

This is the reason why the Japanese, for instance, place such value on a teacup that is crooked or cracked. Because only those things resemble the natural world, only those things that are flawed, incomplete, and transient can truly be beautiful.

Ichi-go ichi-e is a complementary Japanese idea that can be translated as "This moment exists only now and won't come again." It is most frequently heard during social gatherings as a reminder that each interaction, whether with friends, family, or strangers, is special and one-of-a-kind and will never happen again. As a result, we should savor the present and avoid dwelling on the past or the future.

The idea is frequently employed in tea ceremonies, Zen meditation, and Japanese martial arts, all of which emphasize being in the moment.

In the West, we've grown accustomed to the durability of the stone structures and cathedrals of Europe, which occasionally gives us the impression that nothing changes and causes us to lose track of time. Greco-Roman architecture adores symmetry, clean lines, imposing facades, and structures and god statues that endure through the ages.

On the other hand, because Japanese architecture is constructed in the spirit of wabi-sabi, it doesn't attempt to be imposing or perfect. The custom of building with wood assumes that these structures will eventually fall apart and require rebuilding by later generations. The human being and everything we create are accepted as having a limited lifespan in Japanese culture.

For example, the Grand Shrine of Ise has historically undergone reconstruction every 20 years. Preserving customs and traditions, which can endure the test of time better than human-made structures, is more crucial than keeping the building standing for future generations.

The secret is to recognize that some things, like the passage of time and the transient nature of our surroundings, are beyond our control.

Ichi-go ichi-e teaches us to live in the moment and appreciate each gift that life gives us. Finding and pursuing our ikigai is crucial for this reason.

Wabi-sabi teaches us to see beauty in imperfections as a chance for improvement.

Beyond resilience: Antifragility

According to legend, the first time Hercules faced the Hydra, he became discouraged upon learning that by removing one of its heads, two would reappear in its place. If the beast grew stronger with each wound, he would never be able to kill it.

We use the word fragile to describe people, things, and organizations that are weakened when harmed, and the words robust and resilient for things that can withstand harm without weakening, but we don't have a word for things that get stronger when harmed, as Nassim Nicholas Taleb explains in Antifragile: Things That Gain from Disorder (up to a point).

Taleb indicates the term antifragile to describe the kind of power the Hydra of Lerna possessed, to discuss things that grow more resilient after being damaged: Beyond resiliency or robustness is antifragility. The antifragile improves while the resilient resists shocks and remains the same.

Catastrophes and exceptional events provide useful models for the explanation of antifragility. Numerous coastal cities and towns in Japan's Thoku region, including Fukushima, suffered severe damage in 2011 as a reuslt of a tsunami.

When we returned to the affected coast two years after the disaster, we had traveled for hours along deteriorating highways and past empty gas stations before passing through a number of ghost towns, whose streets had been overtaken by the remains of homes, piles of cars, and abandoned train stations. The government had abandoned these towns, which were vulnerable areas unable to recover on their own.

While Ishinomaki and Kesennuma suffered severe damage, they were rebuilt within a few years with the help of many. Ishinomaki and Kesennuma demonstrated their resiliency by being able to carry on as usual in the wake of the disaster.

The Fukushima nuclear power plant was impacted by the tsunami that was brought on by the earthquake. The engineers from Tokyo Electric Power Company who were manning the plant weren't equipped to repair that kind of harm. It will continue to be an emergency for decades at the Fukushima nuclear power plant. As a result of an unprecedented catastrophe, it revealed its vulnerability.

Moments after the earthquake, the Japanese stock markets were closed. Which companies recovered more successfully? The need to rebuild the entirety of the Thoku coast has been good for construction; shares of large construction companies have been steadily rising since 2011.

228

Considering how much they profited from the disaster, Japanese construction companies are in this instance antifragile.

Let's now examine how we can use this idea in our everyday lives. How can we become more resilient?

Step 1: Create redundancies

Try to find a way to earn money from your hobbies, other jobs, or by starting your own business rather than relying solely on one salary. If you only receive one salary, you may be vulnerable if your employer experiences financial difficulties because you may be left with nothing. On the other hand, if you have other employment options and your primary position is lost, it may happen that you end up spending more time at your secondary position and perhaps even earning more money there. In that scenario, you would have overcome your bad luck and would be antifragile.

All of the seniors we spoke with in Ogimi had a primary and a secondary job. The majority of them kept a vegetable garden as a side business and sold their produce at the neighborhood market.

The same is true of personal interests and friendships. It simply involves not putting all of your eggs in one basket, as the saying goes.

There are people who devote their entire attention to their partner and make them their entire world in the context of romantic relationships. If the relationship doesn't work out, those people lose everything, whereas if they've developed strong friendships and a full life along the way, they'll be in a better position to move on after a relationship ends. They'll be antifragile.

Perhaps you are currently thinking, "I don't need more than one salary, and I'm content with the friends I've always had. What's the point of adding something new? Since extraordinary things don't typically occur, it might seem pointless to add variety to our daily activities. We settle into a comfortable place. But sooner or later, the unforeseen always happens.

Step 2: Bet conservatively in certain areas and take many small risks in others

It turns out that the financial industry is very helpful in illuminating this idea. If you have $10,000 in savings, you might invest $9,000 of it in an index fund or fixed-term deposit and the remaining $1,000, say, $100 each in ten start-ups with significant growth potential.

One scenario is that three of the businesses fail (you lose $300), three other businesses' values decrease (you lose another $100 or $200), three other businesses' values increase (you gain $100 or $200), and one of the start-ups' values rise twentyfold (you gain nearly $2,000, or possibly even more).

Even if three of the businesses fail completely, you still make money. Like the Hydra, you've benefited from the damage.

The secret to becoming antifragile is taking on small risks that could result in big rewards while avoiding dangers that could destroy us, like investing $10,000 in a fund with a dubious reputation that we saw advertised in the newspaper.

Step 3: Get rid of the things that make you fragile

For this exercise, we're going the other way. What makes me vulnerable, you might ask? We suffer losses because of the actions, possessions, and habits of some people. Who are they, what are they?

We frequently emphasize taking on new challenges in our lives when we make New Year's resolutions. This kind of goal is great, but establishing "good riddance" goals can have a much greater impact. Consider this:

- Stop snacking between meals
- Eat sweets only once a week
- Gradually pay off all debt
- Avoid spending time with toxic people
- Avoid spending time doing things we don't enjoy, simply because we feel obligated to do them
- Spend no more than twenty minutes on Facebook per day

Adversity should not be feared because it presents an opportunity for growth, so that we can develop resilience in our lives. If we adopt an antifragile mentality, we'll find a way to grow more resilient with each setback, enhancing our way of life and maintaining our attention on our ikigai.

As long as we keep making corrections and establishing new, more ambitious goals, taking a hit or two can be seen as either a misfortune or as a lesson we can apply to every aspect of our lives. "We need randomness, mess, adventures, uncertainty, self-discovery, hear traumatic episodes," writes Taleb in Antifragile. "All these things make life worth living." We recommend reading Nassim Nicholas Taleb's book Antifragile if you're interested in the idea of antifragility.

The wabi-sabi philosophy teaches us that life is pure imperfection and that everything is transient. However, if you have a firm grasp of your ikigai, each moment will be filled with so many possibilities that it will seem to last an eternity.

Conclusion

Each of us has a unique ikigai, but we all seek meaning, and that is something that unites us. We live more fully when we are able to connect with what is important to us throughout the day; when that connection is lost, we experience hopelessness.

Since modern life increasingly distances us from our true selves, it is very simple for us to live meaningless lives. Money, power, attention, success, and other strong forces and incentives constantly divert us; don't let them rule your life.

Intuition and curiosity are two of our most potent internal compass tools for connecting with our ikigai. Follow your passions, abandon your dislikes, or make them your own. Follow your curiosity and keep busy by engaging in activities that bring you joy and meaning. We may find meaning in being good parents or in helping our neighbors; it doesn't have to be a big thing.

To communicate with our ikigai, there is no ideal method. However, we discovered from the Okinawans that we shouldn't stress out too much about finding it.

The ten rules of ikigai

Ten rules that we have gained from the experience of Ogimi's long-living citizens will bring this journey to a close:

Stay active; don't retire. Those who stop doing the things they excel at and enjoy lose their sense of purpose in life. Because of this, it's critical to continue making progress, adding value, enhancing the lives of others, helping others, and influencing the world around you long after your "official" professional activity has ended.

Take it slow. Being in a hurry is inversely proportional to quality of life. As the old saying goes, "Walk slowly and you'll go far." When we leave urgency behind, life and time take on new meaning.

Don't fill your stomach. Less is more when it comes to eating for long life, too. According to the 80 percent rule, in order to stay healthier longer, we should eat a little less than our hunger demands instead of stuffing ourselves.

Surround yourself with good friends. Friends are the best medicine, there for confiding worries over a good chat, sharing stories that brighten your day, getting advice, having fun, dreaming ... in other words, living.

Get in shape for your next birthday. Water flows; it is at its best when it does not stagnate and is free to flow. To keep your body functioning for a very long time, it needs a little daily upkeep. In addition, physical activity causes the release of happy hormones.

Smile. A cheerful attitude is not only relaxing—it also helps make friends. It's good to recognize the things that aren't so great, but we should never forget what a privilege it is to be in the here and now in a world so full of possibilities.

Reconnect with nature. Though most people live in cities these days, human beings are made to be part of the natural world. We should return to it often to recharge our batteries.

Give thanks. To your ancestors, nature, which provides you with the food and air you breathe, your friends and family, and everything else that makes you feel happy and fortunate to be alive. Give thanks for a moment each day, and you'll notice an increase in your happiness.

Live in the moment. Stop regretting the past and fearing the future. Today is all you have. Make the most of it. Make it worth remembering.

Follow your *ikigai*. You have a passion and a special talent inside of you that give your days purpose and inspire you to give your all until the very end. Your goal is to identify your ikigai if you don't already know what it is, as Viktor Frankl once said.

Printed in Great Britain
by Amazon

19387797R00136